C0-BQT-570

Multivariate Interpretation of Clinical Laboratory Data

STATISTICS: Textbooks and Monographs

A SERIES EDITED BY

Vol. 1: The Generalized Jackknife Statistic, *H. L. Gray and W. R. Schucany*
Vol. 2: Multivariate Analysis, *Anant M. Kshirsagar*
Vol. 3: Statistics and Society, *Walter T. Federer*
Vol. 4: Multivariate Analysis: A Selected and Abstracted Bibliography, 1957-1972, *Kocherlakota Subrahmaniam and Kathleen Subrahmaniam* (out of print)
Vol. 5: Design of Experiments: A Realistic Approach, *Virgil L. Anderson and Robert A. McLean*
Vol. 6: Statistical and Mathematical Aspects of Pollution Problems, *John W. Pratt*
Vol. 7: Introduction to Probability and Statistics (in two parts), Part I: Probability; Part II: Statistics, *Narayan C. Giri*
Vol. 8: Statistical Theory of the Analysis of Experimental Designs, *J. Ogawa*
Vol. 9: Statistical Techniques in Simulation (in two parts), *Jack P. C. Kleijnen*
Vol. 10: Data Quality Control and Editing, *Joseph I. Naus* (out of print)
Vol. 11: Cost of Living Index Numbers: Practice, Precision, and Theory, *Kali S. Banerjee*
Vol. 12: Weighing Designs: For Chemistry, Medicine, Economics, Operations Research, Statistics, *Kali S. Banerjee*
Vol. 13: The Search for Oil: Some Statistical Methods and Techniques, *edited by D. B. Owen*
Vol. 14: Sample Size Choice: Charts for Experiments with Linear Models, *Robert E. Odeh and Martin Fox*
Vol. 15: Statistical Methods for Engineers and Scientists, *Robert M. Bethea, Benjamin S. Duran, and Thomas L. Boullion*
Vol. 16: Statistical Quality Control Methods, *Irving W. Burr*
Vol. 17: On the History of Statistics and Probability, *edited by D. B. Owen*
Vol. 18: Econometrics, *Peter Schmidt*
Vol. 19: Sufficient Statistics: Selected Contributions, *Vasant S. Huzurbazar (edited by Anant M. Kshirsagar)*
Vol. 20: Handbook of Statistical Distributions, *Jagdish K. Patel, C. H. Kapadia, and D. B. Owen*
Vol. 21: Case Studies in Sample Design, *A. C. Rosander*
Vol. 22: Pocket Book of Statistical Tables, *compiled by R. E. Odeh, D. B. Owen, Z. W. Birnbaum, and L. Fisher*
Vol. 23: The Information in Contingency Tables, *D. V. Gokhale and Solomon Kullback*
Vol. 24: Statistical Analysis of Reliability and Life-Testing Models: Theory and Methods, *Lee J. Bain*
Vol. 25: Elementary Statistical Quality Control, *Irving W. Burr*
Vol. 26: An Introduction to Probability and Statistics Using BASIC, *Richard A. Groeneveld*

Vol. 27: Basic Applied Statistics, *B. L. Raktoe and J. J. Hubert*
Vol. 28: A Primer in Probability, *Kathleen Subrahmaniam*
Vol. 29: Random Processes: A First Look, *R. Syski*
Vol. 30: Regression Methods: A Tool for Data Analysis, *Rudolf J. Freund and Paul D. Minton*
Vol. 31: Randomization Tests, *Eugene S. Edgington*
Vol. 32: Tables for Normal Tolerance Limits, Sampling Plans, and Screening, *Robert E. Odeh and D. B. Owen*
Vol. 33: Statistical Computing, *William J. Kennedy, Jr. and James E. Gentle*
Vol. 34: Regression Analysis and Its Application: A Data-Oriented Approach, *Richard F. Gunst and Robert L. Mason*
Vol. 35: Scientific Strategies to Save Your Life, *I. D. J. Bross*
Vol. 36: Statistics in the Pharmaceutical Industry, *edited by C. Ralph Buncher and Jia-Yeong Tsay*
Vol. 37: Sampling from a Finite Population, *J. Hajek*
Vol. 38: Statistical Modeling Techniques, *S. S. Shapiro*
Vol. 39: Statistical Theory and Inference in Research, *T. A. Bancroft and C.-P. Han*
Vol. 40: Handbook of the Normal Distribution, *Jagdish K. Patel and Campbell B. Read*
Vol. 41: Recent Advances in Regression Methods, *Hrishikesh D. Vinod and Aman Ullah*
Vol. 42: Acceptance Sampling in Quality Control, *Edward G. Schilling*
Vol. 43: The Randomized Clinical Trial and Therapeutic Decisions, *edited by Niels Tygstrup, John M. Lachin, and Erik Juhl*
Vol. 44: Regression Analysis of Survival Data in Cancer Chemotherapy, *Walter H. Carter, Jr., Galen L. Wampler, and Donald M. Stablein*
Vol. 45: A Course in Linear Models, *Anant M. Kshirsagar*
Vol. 46: Clinical Trials: Issues and Approaches, *edited by Stanley H. Shapiro and Thomas H. Louis*
Vol. 47: Statistical Analysis of DNA Sequence Data, *edited by B. S. Weir*
Vol. 48: Nonlinear Regression Modeling: A Unified Practical Approach, *David A. Ratkowsky*
Vol. 49: Attribute Sampling Plans, Tables of Tests and Confidence Limits for Proportions, *Robert E. Odeh and D. B. Owen*
Vol. 50: Experimental Design, Statistical Models, and Genetic Statistics, *edited by Klaus Hinkelmann*
Vol. 51: Statistical Methods for Cancer Studies, *edited by Richard G. Cornell*
Vol. 52: Practical Statistical Sampling for Auditors, *Arthur J. Wilburn*
Vol. 53: Statistical Signal Processing, *edited by Edward J. Wegman and James G. Smith*
Vol. 54: Self-Organizing Methods in Modeling: GMDH Type Algorithms, *edited by Stanley J. Farlow*
Vol. 55: Applied Factorial and Fractional Designs, *Robert A. McLean and Virgil L. Anderson*
Vol. 56: Design of Experiments: Ranking and Selection, *edited by Thomas J. Santner and Ajit C. Tamhane*
Vol. 57: Statistical Methods for Engineers and Scientists. Second Edition, Revised and Expanded, *Robert M. Bethea, Benjamin S. Duran, and Thomas L. Boullion*
Vol. 58: Ensemble Modeling: Inference from Small-Scale Properties to Large-Scale Systems, *Alan E. Gelfand and Crayton C. Walker*
Vol. 59: Computer Modeling for Business and Industry, *Bruce L. Bowerman and Richard T. O'Connell*
Vol. 60: Bayesian Analysis of Linear Models, *Lyle D. Broemeling*
Vol. 61: Methodological Issues for Health Care Surveys, *Brenda Cox and Steven Cohen*
Vol. 62: Applied Regression Analysis and Experimental Design, *Richard J. Brook and Gregory C. Arnold*

Vol. 63: Statpal: A Statistical Package for Microcomputers – PC-DOS Version for the IBM PC and Compatibles, *Bruce J. Chalmer and David G. Whitmore*
Vol. 64: Statpal: A Statistical Package for Microcomputers – Apple Version for the II, II+, and IIe, *David G. Whitmore and Bruce J. Chalmer*
Vol. 65: Nonparametric Statistical Inference, Second Edition, Revised and Expanded, *Jean Dickinson Gibbons*
Vol. 66: Design and Analysis of Experiments, *Roger G. Petersen*
Vol. 67: Statistical Methods for Pharmaceutical Research Planning, *Sten W. Bergman and John C. Gittins*
Vol. 68: Goodness-of-Fit Techniques, *edited by Ralph B. D'Agostino and Michael A. Stephens*
Vol. 69: Statistical Methods in Discrimination Litigation, *edited by D. H. Kaye and Mikel Aickin*
Vol. 70: Truncated and Censored Samples from Normal Populations, *Helmut Schneider*
Vol. 71: Robust Inference, *M. L. Tiku, W. Y. Tan, and N. Balakrishnan*
Vol. 72: Statistical Image Processing and Graphics, *edited by Edward J. Wegman and Douglas J. DePriest*
Vol. 73: Assignment Methods in Combinatorial Data Analysis, *Lawrence Hubert*
Vol. 74: Econometrics and Structural Change, *Lyle D. Broemeling and Hiroki Tsurumi*
Vol. 75: Multivariate Interpretation of Clinical Laboratory Data, *Adelin Albert and Eugene K. Harris*
Vol. 76: Statistical Tools for Simulation Practitioners, *Jack P. C. Kleijnen*
Vol. 77: Randomization Tests, Second Edition, *Eugene S. Edgington*

OTHER VOLUMES IN PREPARATION

MULTIVARIATE INTERPRETATION OF CLINICAL LABORATORY DATA

Adelin Albert
University of Liège
Liège, Belgium

Eugene K. Harris
University of Virginia
Charlottesville, Virginia

Marcel Dekker, Inc. • New York and Basel

Library of Congress Cataloging in Publication Data

Albert, Adelin
Multivariate interpretation of clinical
laboratory data.

(Statistics, textbooks and monographs ; vol 75)
Includes bibliographies and index.
1. Diagnosis, Laboratory–Statistical methods.
2. Multivariate analysis. I. Harris, Eugene K.,
II. Title. III. Series: Statistics,
textbooks and monographs ; v. 75. [DNLM:
1. Diagnosis, Laboratory. 2. Prognosis.
3. Statistics. QY 25 A333m]
RB38.3.A43 1987 616.07'5 86-25595
ISBN 0-8247-7735-2

MARCEL DEKKER, INC.
270 Madison Avenue, New York, New York 10016

Current printing (last digit) :
10 9 8 7 6 5 4 3 2 1

PRINTED IN THE UNITED STATES OF AMERICA

To Professor Camille Heusghem
Mentor and Friend

Preface

Clinical laboratory tests have long been a routine part of medical examination. An experienced physician becomes adept at integrating test results and other items of information about the patient into a coherent pattern. However, this integrative process, important as it is to the patient's welfare, tends to obscure a rather special characteristic of the laboratory result. More directly than any other piece of information about the patient, the laboratory test represents an amalgam of two basic influences: the patient's own physical state at the time and the biology of the human population to which he or she belongs. Optimal interpretation requires that both effects be taken into account, properly weighted relative to each other. Although this ideal may never be fully achievable, we describe in this book some approaches to it in the form of statistical methods for the analysis of multivariate laboratory data.

The traditional and still popular statistical guideline for interpreting such data is the population-based "reference range." However, applying a separate reference range to each variable in a multivariate set will often, by chance alone, indicate apparent abnormalities, which disappear when the correlations among the variables are accounted for. In Chapter 3, following a brief description in the preceding chapter of multivariate normal distributions, we describe the construction of multivariate reference regions and discuss both advantages and dangers in their use.

Reference regions for laboratory tests are generally based on data from apparently healthy persons. Even when correctly indicating the presence of disease, they offer in themselves little basis for a specific diagnosis. The task of differential diagnosis requires comparable data from patients with the diseases one wants to distinguish. In Chapter 4, we introduce statistical aids to differential diagnosis in the simplest situation: two diagnostic categories, one of which might be a specified disease and the other, different diseases in a given class of pathologies. With respect to kinds of variables, we start with the simplest, a single binary test, including the dichotomized continuous variable. After reviewing the well-known concepts of sensitivity and specificity applicable to this simple case, we show how the likelihood ratio generalizes these concepts to a multivariate set of binary and continuous variables. By selecting an arbitrary cutoff (or "decision") point, this ratio eliminates the need to reduce each continuous variable to binary form.

The next step is to introduce a mathematical model for the likelihood ratio that fits all binary and normally distributed variables and seems also to work well for skewed distributions. This model provides a general statistical tool for summarizing multivariate data to help resolve the problem of distinguishing between two disease categories. We take this further in Chapter 5, discussing the theory and use of multivariate discriminant functions to differentiate three or more diagnostic groups. Both the classical multinormal approach and the more recent logistic discriminant analysis are discussed. Also included are methods to handle the critical tasks of selecting the best variables and assessing the performance of any decision-making aid.

Chapters 6 and 7 are concerned with the use of multivariate analysis in prognosis, the prediction of the future state of the patient based on clinical data and laboratory test results. Chapter 6 considers the case of predicting outcome only at a fixed time in the future after the collection of data has been completed. When only two outcomes are involved, standard discriminant analysis suffices, and we compare logistic and classical "probit" models. The latter postulates a normally distributed underlying, but unobservable, risk of (or susceptibility to) the unfavorable outcome. When more than two outcomes are being considered, one may take advantage of a natural ordering that usually exists among them. Estimation of threshold points and a single linear function of the measured variables turns out to be a simpler predictive technique than estimation of two or more linear discriminant functions.

Often, a series of multivariate observations is available for each patient. In Chapter 6, we propose computation of an average "response curve" for each variable over time among patients in each outcome class. Then, the multivariate "distance" between the response curve of an individual patient and each average curve provides a metric for predicting eventual outcome.

Chapter 7 introduces a "dynamic" approach to prognosis. At each sampling time, a new prediction of outcome during the next time interval is made based on all or part of the data already obtained from that patient. By fitting successive linear models of increasing scope, one can determine which items of recorded clinical and laboratory data are the best short-term predictors. An example based on daily monitoring of patients following myocardial infarction is included. Similar examples, all based on real data, will be found throughout the book.

Continuing to explore the area of dynamic prediction, Chapter 8 discusses various time series models for tracking successive test results from apparently healthy individuals or outpatients. The aim here is not to classify the patient into one or another prognostic group, but simply to detect statistically significant deviations in test values from what would have been expected given the past record of observations. The practical methods are univariate, but current possibilities of multivariate dynamic predictive models are also considered.

Before any of the foregoing, the reader will encounter in Chapter 1 a review of basic probability, the maximum likelihood method of estimation, and operations with vectors and matrices. The primary reason for including this material is to give the reader some flavor for mathematical statistical notation and to define early on some of the terms and concepts used in later chapters. The chapter concludes with a short list of general texts on statistics and multivariate analysis.

The final appendix contains two computer programs to implement some of the methods discussed in the book: a program for multiple group logistic discrimination and a program for analysis of serial, equispaced observations. Other relevant programs, with accompanying instructions for use, are available on request to the authors.

The first author of this book owes thanks to present and past colleagues of the Laboratory of Clinical Chemistry for helpful discussions and much of the illustrative material included. In particular, his indebtedness goes to Professor C. Heusghem under whose stimulating and competent guidance he worked and researched for fifteen years. He is grateful to his former preceptors, Professors H. Breny, M. J. R. Healy, and the late J. A. Anderson, who introduced him to the fascinating world of probability and statistics. Professor Anderson's untimely death in 1983 interrupted a deep friendship and promising collaborative research projects.

The preparation of our book would not have been possible without the invaluable help of Mrs. Janice Lynn Delaval, who typed the entire manuscript with outstanding competence, and of Mrs. Aline De Wulf and Mr. Claude Ernotte, who prepared the artwork.

Adelin Albert
Eugene K. Harris

Contents

1

THE BASICS OF PROBABILITY THEORY AND MATRIX ALGEBRA

1.1
INTRODUCTION

This book is not devoted to statistical theory itself but rather the use of theory to help in interpreting multivariate clinical laboratory data. We shall try, therefore, to limit this chapter to just those theoretical topics necessary for our purpose. The applications of multivariate statistics require a special, compact notation simply to avoid tiresome repetition of symbols when the same operation is applied to each variable. This need is met by adopting vector notation, described below, through which a series of variables, or their observed values, may be represented by a single symbol. Further, since multivariate analysis involves performing the arithmetic operations of addition, subtraction, and multiplication of vectors, both singly and in groups, we need an even more general and compact notation plus a set of rules for carrying out these operations. This is provided by matrix notation, the rules constituting what is called the algebra of vectors and matrices. Again, we shall describe only those elements of this algebra that are essential for our purposes later on.

We also need to review some basic concepts of probability theory, in particular the notion of a random variable and the probability that a random variable will possess a given characteristic. Since readers who are neither statisticians nor mathematicians are more likely to have some acquaintance with the axioms of probability than with the algebra of matrices, we will start with a brief discussion of random variables and probability.

1.2
RANDOM VARIABLES AND PROBABILITIES

The concept of a random variable involves, first of all, the idea of an experiment—a procedure whose results cannot be predicted with certainty. Familiar examples in statistics are the toss of a fair coin or the selection and examination of a group

TABLE 1.1 List of Outcomes and Their Probabilities for the Random Variable: The Sum of Points Appearing on a Roll of Two Fair Dice

Outcome	Probability	Cumulative probability
2	1/36	1/36
3	2/36	3/36
4	3/36	6/36
5	4/36	10/36
6	5/36	15/36
7	6/36	21/36
8	5/36	26/36
9	4/36	30/36
10	3/36	33/36
11	2/36	35/36
12	1/36	36/36 = 1

of subjects. In clinical laboratory work, the experiment usually includes a biochemical method described in detail so that other investigators may repeat the work as closely as possible. Suppose that each such experiment has some object that it produces. For example, the object might be an electrical voltage or some other physical quantity that can be translated to the concentration or activity of a biochemical constituent. In rolling two dice, the object is usually the sum of the points on each face. In these experiments, the objects are called random variables. We associate with any random variable a set of possible outcomes. If numerical (not always the case), these outcomes are called the values the random variable may assume. For example, in a roll of two fair dice, there are eleven possible values, 2, 3, . . . , 12. However, when the object is the future state of a patient, the set of outcomes might be defined to include only the nonnumerical results, full recovery, recovery with disability, or death.

Suppose we consider a certain number of experimental units (or repetitions of the experimental procedure) in which the random variable has been evaluated. Let this number be

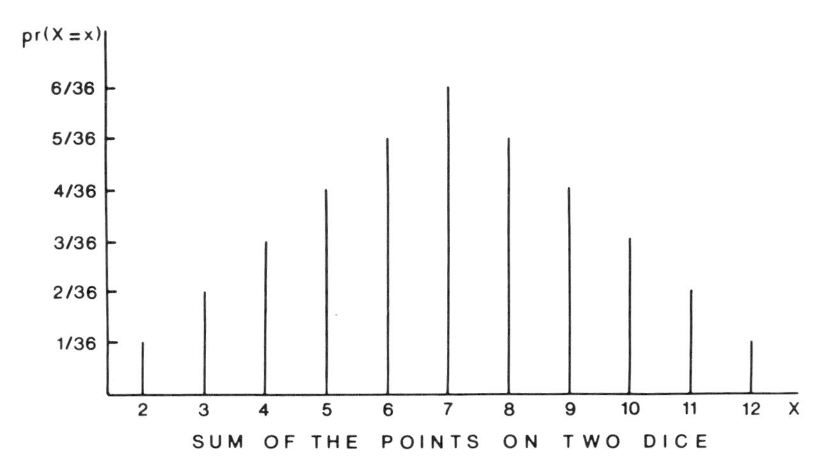

FIGURE 1.1 Distribution of the probabilities that the sum of the points on two dice will take on the value x, after a single roll.

denoted by N, and let $N(O_i)$ denote the subset of N for which the random variable assumed the value (or outcome) O_i. Then, the relative frequency of O_i is defined by $N(O_i)/N$. As N increases, this relative frequency generally settles down close to a theoretical (one may say, ideal) value called the probability of O_i. The "settling down" process is not a uniform one, however; sometimes the relative frequency exactly equals the probability when N is small, only to deviate again at some larger value of N. But as N increases, such deviations tend to get smaller and smaller. In Table 1.1 are shown the probabilities associated with the values of the sum of the faces after a roll of two fair dice. The denominator of each fraction is the total number of faces available when two dice are rolled: for each face of one die, there are six of the other, and all are equally likely to appear. The numerator is the subset of this number yielding the desired sum of points. Taken together, these probabilities form a probability distribution, as in Figure 1.1.

We would run into trouble with this definition of probability if the set of outcomes were infinitely dense, like the points on the real number line. Therefore, later in this chapter we shall generalize this relatively simple definition.

1.3 THE ADDITION RULE FOR MUTUALLY EXCLUSIVE OUTCOMES

Still restricting ourselves to a set of outcomes with integer values (or whole number codes if the outcomes are qualitative classes), let us suppose that this set includes all m possible outcomes of this experiment, and that these are mutually exclusive in the sense that no two can occur in the same experimental unit. Then, two results follow. First, the probability that any one of a subset of $h < m$ outcomes will occur is equal to the sum of the respective probabilities. This is expressed by the equation,

$$\mathrm{pr}(O_1 \text{ or } O_2 \text{ or } \cdots \text{ or } O_h) = \mathrm{pr}(O_1) + \mathrm{pr}(O_2) + \cdots + \mathrm{pr}(O_h)$$

Thus, in rolling two dice, the probability of either a 7 or 11 is $(6/36) + (2/36) = (8/36) = (2/9) = 0.222$.

Second, when $h = m$

$$\mathrm{pr}(O_1 \text{ or } O_2 \cdots \text{ or } O_m) = \mathrm{pr}(O_1) + \cdots + \mathrm{pr}(O_m) = 1 \qquad (1.1)$$

These two equations represent the addition rule in probability theory for mutually exclusive outcomes of integer-valued variables.

1.4 THE MULTIPLICATION RULE

Suppose now that two experiments are performed on each experimental unit. Each experiment has its own object (random variable) associated with a set of possible outcomes (values). For example, the experimental unit might be a patient on whom the first experiment consists of a clinical examination to determine if he or she is suffering from disease D. The random variable is the patient's condition with respect to D. There are two mutually exclusive outcomes: presence of D, labeled simply D, and absence of D, labeled $\overline{D}$. Let the second experiment consist of determining the patient's past exposure to some environmental hazard that might induce D. The random variable here is the degree of exposure, and we postulate three outcomes: minimal or no exposure, moderate exposure, or heavy exposure, labeled S_1, S_2, and S_3, respectively. Assume that each patient can be classified into one of these three outcomes. After performing these two experiments on each of a large group of patients, we ask: What is the probability that a patient in the group possesses both D and S_3? Since these are clearly not mutually exclusive outcomes, the question is not an empty one. Earlier, we defined probability as the limit of a relative frequency as N increases. For simplicity here, we will use the equal sign to mean "limit of," and write

$$\text{pr}(D \text{ and } S_3) = N(D,S_3)/N, \qquad \text{for large } N \tag{1.2}$$

The right side of this equation may be expanded, without changing its numerical value, by multiplying and dividing by $N(D)$, the total number of patients with the disease. Thus, we may write

$$\text{pr}(D \text{ and } S_3) = \left(\frac{N(D)}{N}\right)\left(\frac{N(D,S_3)}{N(D)}\right) \tag{1.3}$$

The second term on the right side is the probability of S_3 among those patients with the disease. It is called the conditional probability of S_3 given D, and is written $\text{pr}(S_3|D)$. Then,

$$\text{pr}(D \text{ and } S_3) = \text{pr}(D)\text{pr}(S_3|D) \tag{1.4}$$

This is an example of the multiplication rule in probability theory, which expresses the probability of the co-existence of two (or more) outcomes in a single experimental unit. Now, if $\mathrm{pr}(S_3|D) = \mathrm{pr}(S_3|\overline{D})$, then the outcome S_3 is said to be independent of the outcomes D or $\overline{D}$. In this case, the conditional probabilities $\mathrm{pr}(S_3|D)$ and $\mathrm{pr}(S_3|\overline{D})$ are equal to the unconditional probability $\mathrm{pr}(S_3)$, which is simply $N(S_3)/N$. Then, the right side of (1.4) becomes just the product of the separate probabilities of the two outcomes, i.e., $\mathrm{pr}(D \text{ and } S_3) = \mathrm{pr}(D)\mathrm{pr}(S_3)$.

The right side of equation (1.2) could equally well have been multiplied by $N(S_3)/N(S_3)$ to give:

$$\mathrm{pr}(D \text{ and } S_3) = \left(\frac{N(S_3)}{N}\right)\left(\frac{N(D,S_3)}{N(S_3)}\right) = \mathrm{pr}(S_3)\mathrm{pr}(D|S_3) \tag{1.5}$$

Equating (1.4) and (1.5),

$$\mathrm{pr}(D)\mathrm{pr}(S_3|D) = \mathrm{pr}(S_3)\mathrm{pr}(D|S_3) \tag{1.6}$$

1.5 BAYES' THEOREM

At this point, using only these basic rules of probability, we can prove the well-known Bayes' theorem at least for two random variables like D and S. From equation (1.6),

$$\mathrm{pr}(D|S_3) = \frac{\mathrm{pr}(D)\mathrm{pr}(S_3|D)}{\mathrm{pr}(S_3)} \tag{1.7}$$

Using both the addition and multiplication laws of probability, $\mathrm{pr}(S_3)$ may be written in the form

$$\mathrm{pr}(S_3) = \mathrm{pr}(D)\mathrm{pr}(S_3|D) + \mathrm{pr}(\overline{D})\mathrm{pr}(S_3|\overline{D})$$

Substituting this expression for $\mathrm{pr}(S_3)$ in equation (1.7),

$$\text{pr}(D|S_3) = \frac{\text{pr}(D)\text{pr}(S_3|D)}{\text{pr}(D)\text{pr}(S_3|D) + \text{pr}(\bar{D})\text{pr}(S_3|\bar{D})} \tag{1.8}$$

This equation is Bayes' theorem for two random variables. The conditional probability $\text{pr}(D|S_3)$ is often called the predictive value of S_3 with respect to the outcome D. A more general appellation for $\text{pr}(D|S_3)$ is the posterior probability of D, in contrast to the unconditional probability $\text{pr}(D)$, called the prior probability of D.

1.6 DEFINITION OF PROBABILITY FOR CONTINUOUS VARIABLES

We mentioned above that defining probability as the limit of the ratio of the number of experimental units for which the random variable assumes a specified value to the total number of units cannot work for variables whose outcomes may be any value on the real number line or even between two points on the real line. Such random variables are called continuous variables, whereas those whose outcomes may be denoted (or coded) by whole numbers are called discrete variables. By definition, the possible values for a continuous variable form an infinitely dense set, so that the probability of a particular value must be zero. On the other hand, no value within the range is impossible. We escape this logical dilemma by noting that although we cannot properly speak of the probability that a continuous variable X will assume a specific value, say x_0, we can consider the probability that any value of X, denoted by x, will not exceed x_0, i.e., the probability that x will fall within a specified range of values.

For a discrete random variable, computing such a probability merely requires summing the probabilities for all values of X up to and including x_0. Suppose, for example, that X is the total number of points appearing after a roll of two dice,

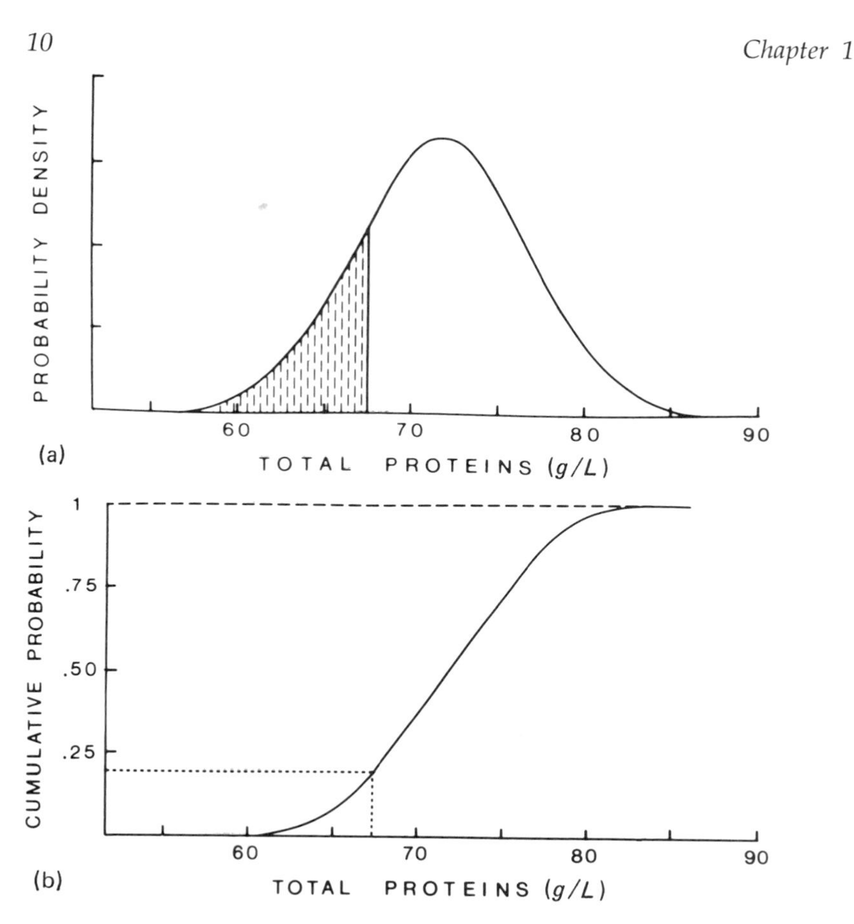

FIGURE 1.2 (a) The probability density function $f(x)$ for the continuous random variable X representing serum total proteins (g/L). (b) The cumulative probability distribution $F(x)$ for the continuous random variable X representing total proteins (g/L).

and x_0 is 7. The column of cumulative probabilities in Table 1.1 tells us that $\mathrm{pr}(X \leq 7)$ equals 21/36, or 7/12.

If X is a continuous variable, the solution is a little more complicated. We have to represent the probability distribution of X by a smooth curve stretching over the range of possible values. An example of such a curve is given in Figure 1.2(a).

Then, the probability we seek is defined as the area under this curve to the left of an ordinate raised at the point x_0, namely, the cross-hatched area in Figure 1.2(a). Calculating this area requires the mathematical operation of integrating the probability distribution represented by the smooth curve between the values minus infinity ($-\infty$) and x_0. When, for reasons of mathematical complexity, the curve cannot be integrated exactly, the area is often found by a procedure called numerical integration, and tables of areas are prepared for closely spaced values x_0 to benefit future users.

It is customary in statistics to designate this smooth curve (or "function") by the symbol $f(x)$. The probability that X does not exceed x_0 would be expressed by the integral,

$$F(x_0) = \text{pr}(X \leq x_0) = \int_{-\infty}^{x_0} f(x)\,dx \tag{1.9}$$

Since $f(x)$ is a probability distribution, it is called a probability density function, or *pdf*, and must satisfy two conditions: (1) $f(x)$ must never be negative; and (2) $F(\infty) = \int_{-\infty}^{\infty} f(x)\,dx$ must equal unity. This last condition, although clearly required by the definition of probability, is still rather remarkable. It says that even if X can assume any value, no matter how large in the negative or positive direction, its cumulative density function $F(\infty)$ over this range must equal one (more precisely, it must be finite even if the range is infinite, because then the reciprocal of this finite value can always be inserted to make the integral unity).

The cumulative density function $F(x)$ derived from the *pdf* in Figure 1.2(a) is shown below it in Figure 1.2(b).

The most famous *pdf* is the normal (or Gaussian) distribution, a bell-shaped curve discussed more fully in the next chapter. The formula representing this *pdf* is

$$f(x) = \frac{1}{\sigma\sqrt{2\pi}} \exp\left\{ -\frac{1}{2}\left(\frac{x-\mu}{\sigma}\right)^2 \right\} \tag{1.10}$$

where "exp(z)" stands for e (e = 2.718 . . . , the base of the natural logarithms) raised to the power z, and μ and σ are special constants called the parameters of the normal distribution. As will be proven in Chapter 2, μ and σ are the mean and standard deviation, respectively, of this distribution, while σ^2 is called the variance. Mathematical proof that the integral of this function from $-\infty$ to $+\infty$ is equal to unity may be found in many textbooks on statistical theory. Although Equation (1.10) is the best known *pdf*, we should remember that all the well-known tests in statistical inference—the t-test, the χ^2-test, the F-test, etc.—involve continuous random variables, each with its own *pdf*, a unique mathematical formula satisfying the two essential conditions of a probability distribution.

In Chapter 2, we discuss the bivariate and multivariate normal distributions as well as the univariate form in Equation (1.10). The great majority of clinical laboratory tests fall naturally into the category of continuous variables, but many clinical signs and symptoms are defined in terms of discrete variables, taking integer values, or classes which may be assigned whole number codes. In addition, the possible diagnostic or prognostic states in a patient may be designated numerically by integers.

Note: For convenience and simplicity, the notation pr(x) will be used throughout this book to refer to the probability distribution of a random variable X. It should be borne in mind, however, that when continuous or a combination of continuous and discrete variables are included in a probability statement, pr(x) actually stands for a density function $f(x)$.

1.7 MAXIMUM LIKELIHOOD ESTIMATION

Probability density functions like the normal distribution are only idealized models of the distributions of large populations of values. In practice, one must deal with relatively small samples of observations. Often it is difficult to define clearly the population from which a particular sample was drawn.

Inevitably, however, the investigator wants to extract general conclusions from his or her data, for example, to derive predictive indices and other statistical tools for classifying new individuals. For this purpose, a descriptive probability model becomes almost essential. Since such a model is characterized by its parameters, statisticians have developed various theories and methods for estimating these parameters from sample data. Today, the most widely accepted and applied theory of estimation is that of maximum likelihood (ML), conceived originally by R. A. Fisher. This method will be referred to often in coming chapters; here we wish only to introduce the procedure and give a couple of simple examples.

Throughout this book, we assume that patients behave independently of each other. Thus, for example, the probability that n_1 patients in a sample have a given disease D while the remaining n_2 patients are nondiseased ($\overline{D}$) will be the product of individual probabilities, in accord with the multiplication rule for independent outcomes. We may express this as

$$\text{pr}(n_1 \in D,\, n_2 \in \overline{D}) = p_{11}\, p_{21} \cdots p_{n_1 1}\, p_{12}\, p_{22} \cdots p_{n_2 2} \qquad (1.11)$$

where the second subscript refers to one of the two disease categories. Now, suppose we hypothesize that all $n_1 + n_2$ patients really represent a set of independent trials, each with the same probability p of disease and $1 - p$ of nondisease. Of course, this hypothesis will almost always be too simplistic, failing to account for differences in ages, environments, etc., but it provides a convenient starting point for the modeling process. We may then condense the product of probabilities on the right-hand side of (1.11) into the simple form, $p^{n_1}(1 - p)^{n_2}$. This (binomial) model is called a likelihood function, or simply a likelihood, of the observed results, and may be denoted by

$$L(p) = p^{n_1}(1 - p)^{n_2} \qquad (1.12)$$

The principle of maximum likelihood instructs us to estimate p as that value which, given the observed numbers n_1 and n_2, maximizes the right-hand side of the likelihood equation (1.12). In practice, it is often more convenient mathematically to find the value of p that maximizes the logarithm of the likelihood. Here,

$$\log L(p) = n_1 \log p + n_2 \log (1 - p)$$

Differentiating the right-hand side with respect to p, setting the derivative equal to zero and solving for p, we obtain the maximum likelihood estimate, $\hat{p} = n_1/(n_1 + n_2)$, not a surprising result. In fact, with no clinical or biochemical information from which to classify a new patient into either the diseased or nondiseased group, the ratio $\hat{p}$ is a natural estimate of the a priori probability of disease, given a training sample of n_1 and n_2 patients. As such information becomes available, the posterior probability for a new patient might differ considerably from $\hat{p}$.

To take a standard textbook example, suppose we hypothesize that a group of sodium measurements from n patients (one per patient) represents a random sample from a single normally distributed population of measurements. The joint likelihood of these observations is

$$L(x_1, x_2, \ldots, x_n) = \prod_{i=1}^{n} \mathrm{pr}(x_i)$$

that is, the product of the individual *pdf*'s. The likelihood function, under the stated hypothesis (or model) is

$$L(\mu, \sigma^2) = (2\pi\sigma^2)^{-n/2} \exp\{(-2\sigma^2)^{-1} \sum_{i=1}^{n} (x_i - \mu)^2\} \qquad (1.13)$$

For any given sample of size n, the expression (1.13) is only a function of the parameters μ and σ^2. The *ML* estimate of σ^2 may be found by differentiating

$$\log L = (-n/2)(\log 2\pi + \log \sigma^2) - (2\sigma^2)^{-1} \sum_{i=1}^{n} (x_i - \mu)^2$$

with respect to σ^2 and setting the derivative to zero, obtaining

$$\hat{\sigma}^2 = (1/n) \sum_{i=1}^{n} (x_i - \mu)^2$$

the average squared deviation from the mean μ. Since in general μ is unknown, its *ML* estimate, the sample mean $\bar{x}$, is substituted. To compensate, the "degrees of freedom" n in the denominator is reduced by one, and the estimate

$$s^2 = \sum_{i=1}^{n} (x_i - \bar{x})^2/(n - 1)$$

is used in place of $\hat{\sigma}^2$. Thus, the "sample variance" s^2 is not an *ML* estimate of the parameter σ^2 in the normal distribution but the best available approximation to it.

In many practical problems, including most of those encountered in this book, the likelihood function is too complicated, even in its logarithmic form, to admit a direct, exact solution for the *ML* estimate. Instead, an iterative procedure embedded in a computer program must be used. This requires a reasonable initial guess of the value of the parameter and the exercise of some care to assure that the final estimate is derived from the true maximum of the likelihood function, not just a local maximum over a limited range of possible values of the parameter.

The maximum likelihood estimate of a parameter of a distribution has been proven to have at least as small a sampling variability as any other possible estimate over repeated random samples from the distribution.

1.8 VECTORS

A. Definition

A laboratory profile is a collection of laboratory tests $X_1, \ldots, X_k$, treated here as random variables. In mathematical notation, such a profile defines a vector, customarily represented by an uppercase boldface letter,

$$\mathbf{X} = \begin{bmatrix} X_1 \\ \vdots \\ X_k \end{bmatrix}$$

The number k defines the dimension of the vector. The vector of observed values is noted with a lowercase letter $\mathbf{x}$. Thus, by definition a vector is always a "column vector" and $X_1, \ldots, X_k$, or $x_1, \ldots, x_k$ are its elements or components. For convenience but also for algebraic purposes, the notation

$$\mathbf{X}^T = (X_1, \ldots, X_k)$$

is used to represent the same vector transposed. Thus, $\mathbf{X}^T$ always signifies a "row vector." For example, in Chapter 3, we take the vector $\mathbf{X}^T = (X_1, X_2, X_3)$ to signify the three-test profile consisting of urea (X_1), uric acid (X_2), and creatinine (X_3). A patient with 5.4 mmol/L of urea, 298 µmol/L of uric acid and 78 μmol/L of creatinine is characterized by the vector $\mathbf{x}^T = (5.4,298,78)$.

B. Vector Operations

Vectors can be added, subtracted, or averaged just as ordinary variables. For example, the addition of two vectors, **X** and **Y**, is obtained by adding the corresponding elements

$$\begin{aligned}\mathbf{X}^T + \mathbf{Y}^T &= (X_1, \ldots, X_k) + (Y_1, \ldots, Y_k) \\ &= (X_1 + Y_1, \ldots, X_k + Y_k) \\ &= (\mathbf{X} + \mathbf{Y})^T\end{aligned}$$

If $\mathbf{x}_1, \ldots, \mathbf{x}_n$ denote the observations of profile **X** on n individuals, the average (or mean) vector is given by

$$\bar{\mathbf{x}} = \frac{1}{n}(\mathbf{x}_1 + \cdots + \mathbf{x}_n) = \frac{1}{n}\sum_{i=1}^{n} \mathbf{x}_i$$

introducing the conventional summation symbol Σ.

Consider the two vectors $\mathbf{x}^T = (1,3,4)$ and $\mathbf{y}^T = (0,1,2)$. Then,

$$\begin{aligned}\mathbf{x}^T + \mathbf{y}^T &= (1 + 0, 3 + 1, 4 + 2) = (1,4,6) \\ \mathbf{x}^T - \mathbf{y}^T &= (1 - 0, 3 - 1, 4 - 2) = (1,2,2)\end{aligned}$$

A single number can be thought of as a vector with only one element, and is called a *scalar*. Multiplication of a vector by a scalar is performed by multiplying each component by the scalar; thus,

$$4\mathbf{x}^T = (4 \times 1, 4 \times 3, 4 \times 4) = (4,12,16)$$

If **X** and **Y** are vectors, the "row by column" product of the two vectors, also called the "inner product," is a scalar. That is,

$$\mathbf{X}^T\mathbf{Y} = x_1y_1 + \cdots + x_ky_k = \sum_{i=1}^{k} x_iy_i, \qquad \text{a single number}$$

For the two vectors **x** and **y** above, the inner product is 11. Inner products are widely used in multivariate statistics to ease the notation. For instance, the linear combination of k variables $X_1, \ldots, X_k$, namely, $a_1X_1 + \cdots + a_kX_k$, can also be written in the shorthand notation $\mathbf{a}^\mathrm{T}\mathbf{X}$, where $\mathbf{a}^\mathrm{T} = (a_1, \ldots, a_k)$ is the row vector of coefficients and **X**, the vector of variables.

1.9 MATRICES

A. Definition

By definition, a matrix is a rectangular array of numbers, called elements, consisting of r rows and c columns:

$$\mathbf{A} = \begin{bmatrix} a_{11} & \cdots & a_{1c} \\ \vdots & & \vdots \\ a_{r1} & \cdots & a_{rc} \end{bmatrix}$$

For example, when observations of a vector $\mathbf{X}^T = (X_1, \ldots, X_k)$ of k variables are available from n subjects, they form a matrix of n rows (subjects) and k columns (variables). Of course, any vector **X** is a matrix with k rows and 1 column, and any scalar a 1×1 matrix.

Matrix dimensions are referred to as $r \times c$. A matrix with the same number of rows as columns is called a square matrix. Matrices are generally denoted by boldface uppercase letters, e.g., **A**, **B**, **X**, etc. The (i,j)th element of a matrix **A** is the element at the intersection of the ith row and jth column; it is written $(\mathbf{A})_{ij}$ or simply a_{ij}.

The transpose of a matrix **A**, written $\mathbf{A}^T$, is obtained by permuting its rows and columns. Thus the transpose of the matrix **A** above is

$$\mathbf{A}^T = \begin{bmatrix} a_{11} & \cdots & a_{r1} \\ \vdots & & \vdots \\ a_{1c} & \cdots & a_{rc} \end{bmatrix}$$

B. Matrix Algebra

Matrices can be added or subtracted like ordinary numbers or vectors, but they must be of equal dimensions. If **A** and **B** are such matrices, then $\mathbf{A} + \mathbf{B}$ and $\mathbf{A} - \mathbf{B}$ are the matrices obtained by respectively adding and subtracting the corresponding elements of **A** and **B**. Multiplication of a matrix by a scalar is carried out by multiplying each element of the matrix by the scalar.

As an example, consider the two matrices:

$$\mathbf{A} = \begin{bmatrix} 1 & 0 & 2 \\ 3 & 5 & 1 \\ 2 & 1 & 0 \end{bmatrix} \quad \mathbf{B} = \begin{bmatrix} 1 & 1 & 2 \\ 0 & 0 & 1 \\ 5 & 2 & 1 \end{bmatrix}$$

Then,

$$\mathbf{A} + \mathbf{B} = \begin{bmatrix} 2 & 1 & 4 \\ 3 & 5 & 2 \\ 7 & 3 & 1 \end{bmatrix}$$

$$\mathbf{A} - \mathbf{B} = \begin{bmatrix} 0 & -1 & 0 \\ 3 & 5 & 0 \\ -3 & -1 & -1 \end{bmatrix}$$

Two matrices can be multiplied if the number of columns in the first matrix equals the number of rows in the second.

Matrices are multiplied "rows by columns"; that is, if **A** is an $m \times k$ matrix and **B** a $k \times n$ matrix, then the product **AB** is an $m \times n$ matrix, whose (i,j)th element is given by

$$(\mathbf{AB})_{ij} = a_{i1}b_{1j} + \cdots + a_{ik}b_{kj} = \sum_{h=1}^{k} a_{ih}b_{hj}$$

Note, however, that the product **BA** cannot be obtained (assuming $m \neq n$). Moreover, if $m = n$, the product **BA** would not be the same matrix as **AB**. This would be true even if both **A** and **B** were square $k \times k$ matrices. In general, matrix multiplication is not commutable like the multiplication of two numbers. An exception to this rule is the multiplication of a matrix by its inverse, defined in subsection C.

The product of the two matrices **A** and **B** is

$$\mathbf{AB} = \begin{bmatrix} 1 & 0 & 2 \\ 3 & 5 & 1 \\ 2 & 1 & 0 \end{bmatrix} \begin{bmatrix} 1 & 1 & 2 \\ 0 & 0 & 1 \\ 5 & 2 & 1 \end{bmatrix} = \begin{bmatrix} 11 & 5 & 4 \\ 8 & 5 & 12 \\ 2 & 2 & 5 \end{bmatrix}$$

We mentioned above that the row by column multiplication of two vectors (i.e., $\mathbf{X}^T\mathbf{Y}$) produced a scalar. However, the column by row product of two vectors yields a matrix. For example, using the vectors $\mathbf{x}^T = (1,3,4)$ and $\mathbf{y}^T = (0,1,2,)$, we found that $\mathbf{x}^T\mathbf{y} = 11$. However,

$$\mathbf{xy}^T = \begin{bmatrix} 1\times0 & 1\times1 & 1\times2 \\ 3\times0 & 3\times1 & 3\times2 \\ 4\times0 & 4\times1 & 4\times2 \end{bmatrix} = \begin{bmatrix} 0 & 1 & 2 \\ 0 & 3 & 6 \\ 0 & 4 & 8 \end{bmatrix}$$

A matrix **S** is said to be symmetric if $\mathbf{S} = \mathbf{S}^T$. This means that all elements above the main diagonal are equal to the corresponding elements below the diagonal, or

$$s_{ij} = s_{ji} \qquad \text{for all } i \text{ and } j$$

For instance, the matrix below is symmetric:

$$\mathbf{S} = \begin{bmatrix} 1 & 5 & 0 \\ 5 & 2 & 3 \\ 0 & 3 & 1 \end{bmatrix}$$

In statistics, many matrices are both square and symmetric. An example particularly important in multivariate analysis is the variance–covariance matrix, defined in Chapter 2.

C. Inverse and Determinant of a Square Matrix

Certain matrix operations, important in multivariate analysis, can be carried out only on square matrices. One of these operations is *inverting* a matrix. The inverse of a square matrix $\mathbf{A}$ is another square matrix denoted by $\mathbf{A}^{-1}$, for which the product $\mathbf{AA}^{-1} = \mathbf{A}^{-1}\mathbf{A} = \mathbf{I}$, where $\mathbf{I}$ represents the *identity matrix* whose elements are all unity along the main diagonal and zero everywhere else. Inversion is the matrix analogue of scalar division. The inverse of a symmetric matrix is also symmetric. Calculating the inverse of any $k \times k$ matrix for which k exceeds three or four is a very time-consuming exercise, but fortunately there now exist many computer programs that will perform this operation quickly and accurately for any reasonably sized matrix.

Matrix inversion involves calculating another quantity associated only with square matrices called the determinant of a matrix. This is denoted by the absolute number symbol, i.e., $|\mathbf{A}|$ represents the determinant of the square matrix $\mathbf{A}$. When $|\mathbf{A}| = 0$, inversion is not possible and the matrix $\mathbf{A}$ is said to be singular. We will not go into the general mathematics of calculating the inverse and determinant of a matrix but will give the formulas for the case when $k = 2$, as in the bivariate normal distribution discussed in the next chapter. In this simplest of cases,

$$|\mathbf{A}| = a_{11}a_{22} - a_{12}a_{21}$$

a scalar as is true for all determinants, while

$$\mathbf{A}^{-1} = \frac{1}{|\mathbf{A}|}\begin{bmatrix} a_{22} & -a_{12} \\ -a_{21} & a_{11} \end{bmatrix}$$

The reader may enjoy verifying that $\mathbf{AA}^{-1} = \mathbf{I}$.

D. Quadratic Forms

The triple product $\mathbf{X}^T\mathbf{SX}$, where $\mathbf{X}$ is a vector and $\mathbf{S}$ a symmetric matrix is called a quadratic form,

$$\mathbf{X}^T\mathbf{SX} = \sum_{i=1}^{k} \sum_{j=1}^{k} s_{ij}X_iX_j$$

For example, when $k = 3$

$$\mathbf{X}^T\mathbf{SX} = s_{11}X_1^2 + s_{22}X_2^2 + s_{33}X_3^2 + 2s_{12}X_1X_2 + 2s_{13}X_1X_3 + 2s_{23}X_2X_3$$

Quadratic forms will be referred to several times in this book, especially when dealing with multivariate distances.

For instance, using the matrix $\mathbf{S}$ above and the vector $\mathbf{x}^T = (1,3,4)$, we have

$$\mathbf{x}^T\mathbf{Sx} = (1,3,4)\begin{bmatrix} 1 & 5 & 0 \\ 5 & 2 & 3 \\ 0 & 3 & 1 \end{bmatrix}\begin{bmatrix} 1 \\ 3 \\ 4 \end{bmatrix}$$

$$= (16,23,13)\begin{bmatrix} 1 \\ 3 \\ 4 \end{bmatrix}$$

$$= 16 \times 1 + 23 \times 3 + 13 \times 4 = 137$$

GENERAL REFERENCE TEXTBOOKS

Armitage, P. (1971). *Statistical Methods in Medical Research*. Blackwell Scientific Publications, Oxford.

Dixon, W. J., and Massey, F. J. (1969). *Introduction to Statistical Analysis*. McGraw-Hill, New York.

Maxwell, A. E. (1977). *Multivariate Analysis in Behavioral Research*. Chapman & Hall, London.

Morrison, D. F. (1976). *Multivariate Statistical Methods*, Chapters 1 and 2. McGraw-Hill, Kogakusha, Tokyo.

Rao, C. R. (1952). *Advanced Statistical Methods in Biometric Research*. Wiley, New York.

Rohatgi, V. J. (1984). *Statistical Inference*. Wiley, New York.

Seal, H. L. (1968). *Multivariate Statistical Analysis for Biologists*. Methuen, London.

Seber, G. A. F. (1984). *Multivariate Observations*. Wiley, New York.

Snedecor, G. E., and Cochran, W. G. (1967). *Statistical Methods*. Iowa State University Press, Ames.

Van de Geer, J. P. (1971). *Introduction to Multivariate Analysis for the Social Sciences*, Chapters 1 to 4. Freeman, San Francisco.

2

Normal Distribution: Univariate–Multivariate

2.1
INTRODUCTION

We turn our attention now to the normal (Gaussian) probability distribution in its univariate, bivariate, and multivariate forms. Although some of the methods discussed in later chapters are quite robust (that is, able to deal successfully with variables of many different distributions), the normal distribution is still of fundamental importance. For example, the assumption of multivariate normality underlies the classical theory of discriminant analysis. Statistical tests of hypotheses about the origins or nature of a set of observations are often based on the normal distribution. Normally distributed variables have the unique property that sample estimates of their means and standard deviations form independent distributions, an important factor in the theory of testing statistical hypotheses. Among the other advantages of the normal distribution is the fact that most scientific workers are familiar with published tables of the univariate normal and with such common statistical tests as Student's "t" and chi-square in its various forms, all derived from this distribution.

Although this book is concerned primarily with the analysis and interpretation of multivariate data, we start with a review of the univariate normal because a set of variables ($X_1, \ldots, X_k$) cannot jointly form a multivariate normal distribution unless each individual variable is normally distributed. Following our description of univariate, bivariate, and multivariate normal distributions, we examine some modern methods for detecting "outliers" in the dataset which, if not separated out, may exert highly disproportionate effects on the results of statistical analysis. Multivariate distributions may require different, more elaborate schemes for outlier detection than those satisfactory for univariate distributions, but we shall also mention a technique that avoids such complications by converting a multivariate index to univariate form.

Finally, we consider some useful current methods for

transforming variables from nonnormal to normally distributed forms, that is, converting their original measurement scales to new ones on which the resulting data will be normally distributed. Of course, it would be convenient if a single transformation scheme could work for all the variables in a multivariate set whose original measurement scales produced nonnormal observations. This will rarely happen and, in any case, is not at all necessary.

2.2
THE UNIVARIATE NORMAL

Although the univariate normal distribution is undoubtedly the most well-known probability distribution, its usefulness in statistics does not arise because it fits the distribution of many naturally observed variables. In fact, it usually does not. Its practical importance is due instead to its convenient mathematical properties with the result that many techniques of statistical analysis assume the existence of normally distributed variables. Even more significant is its central role in the general development of statistics as a mathematical science. This is exemplified by the central limit theorem, which states, for practical purposes, that the distribution of means of random samples of size n from a population tends more and more to the normal form as n increases regardless of the form of the original distribution (for $n = 1$). The only condition is that the parent population possesses a finite variance.

A random variable X is normally distributed if it meets the following conditions:

a. X is a continuous variable that may assume any value x along the axis of real numbers from $-\infty$ (infinitely distant from zero in the negative direction) to $+\infty$ (infinitely distant from zero in the positive direction).

b. The probability distribution of the values of X, denoted by $\text{pr}(x)$, conforms to the symmetrical bell-shaped curve

$$\text{pr}(x) = (2\pi\sigma^2)^{-1/2} \exp\left\{ -\frac{1}{2} \frac{(x - \mu)^2}{\sigma^2} \right\} \qquad -\infty < x < +\infty \tag{2.1}$$

As noted in Chapter 1 and proven in the appendix to this chapter, the parameter μ is the mean of the values of X, σ is their standard deviation, and σ^2 the variance of those values. The probability that X will assume values within the range of numbers a to b may be obtained by integrating the right-hand side of equation (2.1) over this range. That is,

$$\text{pr}(a \leq X \leq b) = \int_a^b (2\pi\sigma^2)^{-1/2} \exp\left\{ -\frac{1}{2} \frac{(x - \mu)^2}{\sigma^2} \right\} dx \tag{2.2}$$

Remarkably, as point a moves leftward towards $-\infty$, and b moves rightward towards $+\infty$, the integral on the right-hand side of equation (2.2) approaches unity while remaining always positive, thus fulfilling the conditions of a probability distribution. However, for all finite values of a and b, the exact value of this integral cannot be obtained mathematically but can only be approximated (albeit to any desired accuracy), for example by series expansion. Such values (areas under the normal curve) are given in the familiar standard normal tables in terms of "standard normal deviates" $z = (x - \mu)/\sigma$.

The univariate normal probability distribution is pictured in Figure 2.1 with σ marked off as a distance from the mean on the x-axis. The area under the normal curve between the points $(\mu - \sigma)$ and $(\mu + \sigma)$, the probability that X will assume a value, $(\mu - \sigma) \leq x \leq (\mu + \sigma)$, is about 0.68, or 68%, while the probability that X will assume a value between $(\mu - 2\sigma)$ and $(\mu + 2\sigma)$ is about 95%.

If the standard deviation of observed values of X in a population is small relative to the mean, then X may appear to be normally distributed even though negative values are

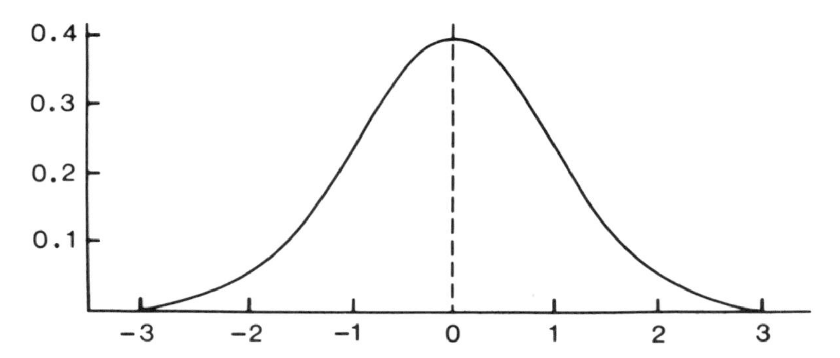

FIGURE 2.1 Univariate normal probability density function.

impossible. This situation often occurs in measurements of such well-controlled variables as serum sodium or calcium. If the standard deviation is large, relative to the mean, the distribution curve will often be skewed to the right, rising rapidly in the lower range of values but then declining slowly to a long tail of high values. Such asymmetry will be much more likely in a biochemical variable whose measurement is less precise at higher values than at lower values. However, the observations can often be reduced to a normal distribution by transforming them to a different measurement scale (e.g., log x). We will review such "normalizing" transformations towards the end of this chapter.

2.3 THE BIVARIATE NORMAL

The multivariate normal distribution is a probability distribution (or "density") function that describes the joint variability shown by two or more normally distributed variables. We discuss first the simplest form of multivariate normal distribution, the bivariate normal. If X and Y are each normally distributed variables with means μ_x,μ_y, standard deviations σ_x,σ_y, respectively, and correlation coefficient ρ, their joint

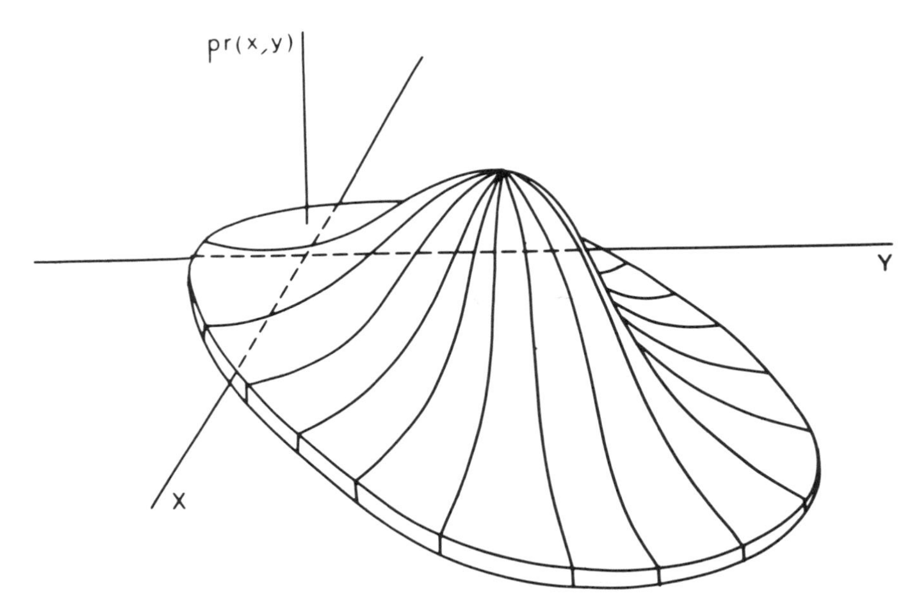

FIGURE 2.2 Bivariate normal probability density function (Mood, 1950).

distribution will generally follow the bivariate normal form, defined as

$$\mathrm{pr}(x,y) = (2\pi\sigma_x\sigma_y\sqrt{1-\rho^2})^{-1} \exp\left[-{}^1\!/_2(1-\rho^2)^{-1}\left\{\frac{(x-\mu_x)^2}{\sigma_x^2} + \frac{(y-\mu_y)^2}{\sigma_y^2} - 2\rho\frac{(x-\mu_x)(y-\mu_y)}{\sigma_x\sigma_y}\right\}\right] \tag{2.3}$$

This equation defines a bell-shaped surface, $z = \mathrm{pr}(x,y)$ as drawn in Figure 2.2. Any plane parallel to the (x,y) plane (i.e., at a fixed value of z), cuts the surface in an elliptical curve which may be expressed as

$$(1-\rho^2)^{-1}\left\{\frac{(x-\mu_x)^2}{\sigma_x^2} + \frac{(y-\mu_y)^2}{\sigma_y^2} - 2\rho\frac{(x-\mu_x)(y-\mu_y)}{\sigma_x\sigma_y}\right\} = K, \text{ a constant} \tag{2.4}$$

Planes perpendicular to the (x,y) plane (i.e., fixed y, random values of X, or fixed x, random values of Y) cut the surface in univariate normal distributions called conditional distributions, $\mathrm{pr}(x|y)$ and $\mathrm{pr}(y|x)$, respectively. The properties of these distributions are described in many statistical texts (e.g., Dixon and Massey, 1969) but are not germane to the subject here.

The correlation coefficient ρ may be defined in both algebraic and geometric terms. First, we recall that the variance of X, σ_x^2, is the expected or mean value of squared deviations $(x - \mu_x)^2$. Similarly, the variance of Y, σ_y^2, is the expected value of $(y - \mu_y)^2$. Now, the expected value of the product of joint deviations $(x - \mu_x)(y - \mu_y)$ is called the covariance of X and Y, say σ_{xy}. The correlation ρ is defined algebraically as the ratio of the covariance to the square root of the product of the two variances; that is, $\rho = \sigma_{xy}/\sigma_x\sigma_y$. The value of the coefficient lies between -1 and $+1$, reaching its absolute maximum value when one variable is strictly proportional to the other, e.g., $y = cx$, for all values of X. When $c = -1$, Y and X are inversely proportional, and $\rho = -1$. When the size of any random deviation $(x - \mu_x)$ is entirely unaffected by the size of the corresponding deviation $(y - \mu_y)$, the covariance and, therefore, the correlation coefficient become zero. In this case, it may be seen from equation (2.3) that the bivariate normal density function reduces to the product of two univariate normal distributions. Uncorrelated normal variables are thus independent of each other in the probability sense.

A geometric intepretation of ρ may be obtained by referring to the ellipse that a plane parallel to the (x,y) plane defines when it cuts the bivariate normal surface. Projecting this ellipse to the (x,y) plane, its major axis will make an angle

$$\theta = \frac{1}{2}\tan^{-1}\left\{\frac{2\rho\sigma_x\sigma_y}{\sigma_x^2 - \sigma_y^2}\right\}$$

with the horizontal (x) axis. Then, when the variables are positively corrrelated $(\rho > 0)$, $0 < \theta < 90°$, and the major axis

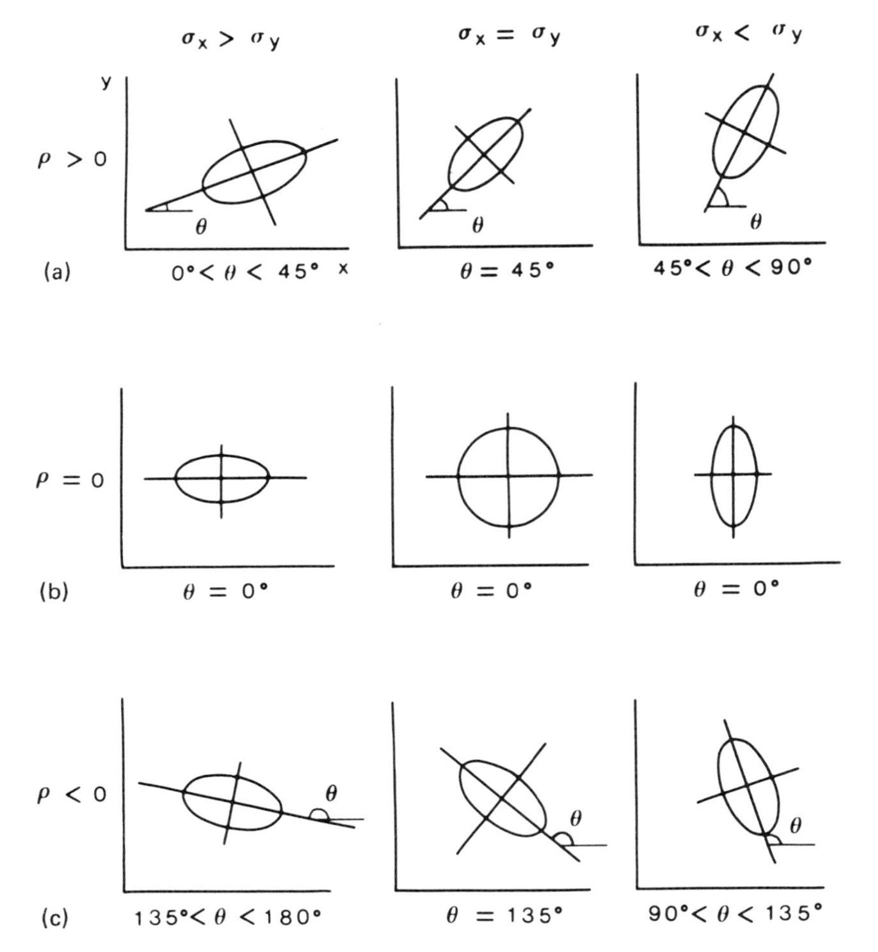

FIGURE 2.3 Contours of equal density of bivariate normal distributions (Johnson and Kotz, 1972).

will tilt in a generally SW to NE direction, as shown in the (a) row of Figure 2.3. When $\rho = 0$, $\theta = 0°$, and the major axis lies either parallel or perpendicular to the x-axis. In this case, when $\sigma_x = \sigma_y$, the ellipse becomes a circle [see the (b) row]. When the variables are negatively correlated ($\rho < 0$), $90° < \theta < 180°$, and the major axis of the ellipse will tilt in a generally NW to SE direction, as shown in the (c) row.

Suppose that all the ellipses generated by passing planes through the bell-shaped bivariate normal surface at different fixed values of z are projected onto the (x,y) plane. They will then form a nest of concentric ellipses, each of which contains a certain proportion of the universe of (x,y) pairs. The ellipse containing 50% of such paired values will lie within the ellipse containing 70%, which will, in turn, lie inside that containing 95%. In terms familiar to the clinical laboratory, each ellipse becomes a bivariate "reference region" for paired values of two tests normally distributed across some defined population of individuals. That is, each ellipse includes a specific percentage, say $(100\,P)$%, of the observations (pairs of values) in the joint distribution of X and Y.

How can we determine the equation of the ellipse corresponding to a given P-value? In statistical theory, the left-hand side of equation (2.4) is called a quadratic form in two variables, and is distributed in a chi-square distribution with 2 degrees of freedom (χ_2^2). Therefore, setting K in equation (2.4) equal to $\chi^2(P;2)$ the Pth percentile of χ_2^2 (e.g., the 95th percentile of χ_2^2 is 5.99), we obtain the equation for the boundary of the desired bivariate region. The ellipse itself may be constructed by selecting a series of x-values and solving the equation for the corresponding y's. Unfortunately, this does not solve the problem in practice because we generally do not know the true means and variances but can only estimate them from a random sample of (x,y) pairs. We shall postpone further discussion of this problem until the next chapter, which is devoted entirely to the calculation and the properties of both univariate and multivariate normal reference regions.

2.4
THE MULTIVARIATE NORMAL

We turn now to a description of the general multivariate normal in $k \geq 2$ variables.

This distribution involves k means, k variances and $k(k - 1)/2$ covariances. Denoting the variables by $X_1, \ldots, X_k$, their variances by $\sigma_{11}, \ldots, \sigma_{kk}$, and covariances by $\sigma_{12}, \sigma_{13}, \ldots, \sigma_{k-1,k}$, we shall represent by $\mathbf{\Sigma}$ a variance–covariance matrix with elements,

$$\mathbf{\Sigma} = \begin{bmatrix} \sigma_{11} & \sigma_{12} & \cdots & \sigma_{1k} \\ \sigma_{21} & \sigma_{22} & \cdots & \sigma_{2k} \\ \vdots & \vdots & & \vdots \\ \sigma_{k1} & \sigma_{k2} & \cdots & \sigma_{kk} \end{bmatrix}$$

Since $\sigma_{ij} = \sigma_{ji}$, the matrix is symmetrical, and only the upper (or lower) triangle need be written down. The multivariate normal distribution (Anderson, 1958; Morrison, 1976) may be written

$$\text{pr}(x_1, \ldots, x_k) = (2\pi)^{-k/2}|\mathbf{\Sigma}|^{-1/2} \exp\left\{ -\frac{1}{2} \sum_{i=1}^{k} \sum_{j=1}^{k} \sigma^{ij}(x_i - \mu_i)(x_j - \mu_j) \right\}$$

where σ^{ij} is the (i,j)th element of the inverse matrix $\mathbf{\Sigma}^{-1}$, and $|\mathbf{\Sigma}|$ is the determinant of the matrix. In matrix notation, letting $\mathbf{x}^T = (x_1, \ldots, x_k)$ and $\boldsymbol{\mu}^T = (\mu_1, \ldots, \mu_k)$, the last equation becomes

$$\text{pr}(\mathbf{x}) = (2\pi)^{-k/2}|\mathbf{\Sigma}|^{-1/2} \exp\{-\frac{1}{2}(\mathbf{x} - \boldsymbol{\mu})^T\mathbf{\Sigma}^{-1}(\mathbf{x} - \boldsymbol{\mu})\} \tag{2.5}$$

For example, the variance-covariance matrix in the bivariate case is

$$\boldsymbol{\Sigma} = \begin{bmatrix} \sigma_x^2 & \rho\sigma_x\sigma_y \\ \rho\sigma_x\sigma_y & \sigma_y^2 \end{bmatrix}$$

with inverse

$$\boldsymbol{\Sigma}^{-1} = \begin{bmatrix} \dfrac{1}{\sigma_x^2(1 - \rho^2)} & \dfrac{-\rho}{\sigma_x\sigma_y(1 - \rho^2)} \\ \dfrac{-\rho}{\sigma_x\sigma_y(1 - \rho^2)} & \dfrac{1}{\sigma_y^2(1 - \rho^2)} \end{bmatrix}$$

The determinant of the matrix is

$$|\boldsymbol{\Sigma}| = \sigma_x^2\sigma_y^2(1 - \rho^2)$$

Substituting these results into equation (2.5) returns us to the bivariate normal density function as expressed in equation (2.3). For our purposes, the multivariate normal may be written more compactly in the form

$$\text{pr}(x_1, \ldots, x_k) = C_k \exp(-Q_k/2) \tag{2.6}$$

where

$$C_k = (2\pi)^{-k/2}|\boldsymbol{\Sigma}|^{-1/2} \quad \text{and} \quad Q_k = (\mathbf{x} - \boldsymbol{\mu})^T \boldsymbol{\Sigma}^{-1} (\mathbf{x} - \boldsymbol{\mu}) \tag{2.7}$$

is a quadratic form distributed as chi-square with k degrees of freedom (χ_k^2).

Setting Q_k equal to a specified percentile of the distribution of χ_k^2 yields the formula for a "hyper-ellipsoidal" region in k-dimensional space, which contains that percentage of the k-variable observation vectors comprising the multivariate normal distribution. As shown in the next chapter, this procedure may be used to derive a multivariate reference region, but only when estimates of the means, variances, and covariances are available from a relatively large random sample, say at least twenty times as many observation vectors as measured variables. When the sample size is smaller than this, more exact methods are needed. However, the statistic $\hat{Q}_k$ can still serve a very useful purpose, testing the assumption that such a sample of observation vectors does indeed come from a multivariate normal distribution. Healy (1968) has suggested plotting the square roots or cube roots of sample values of $\hat{Q}_k$ on normal probability paper. He reasons that the points should plot more or less linearly if the underlying distribution is multivariate normal because, even for small values of k, the distribution of the root of a χ_k^2 variable is closely approximated by a standard normal distribution.*

We consider now a problem that always arises when we are trying to summarize a collection of measurements obtained from many individuals. How do we detect outliers, observations that come from distributions different from that of the great majority of observed values? Our primary purpose, if we find such observations, should be to ascertain why they came to differ so markedly from their fellows. Often, no clear reason can be found. In any case, real outliers, which by definition are relatively rare events, must be set aside at least temporarily so that summary statistics like means, variances, and reference regions may be derived from a reasonably homogeneous set of observations.

2.5 DETECTION OF OUTLIERS IN MULTIVARIATE NORMAL POPULATIONS

Barnett and Lewis's recent book (1978) provides a valuable guide to methods for detecting outliers in multivariate samples. Labeling one or more observation vectors as "outliers"

---

*Healy's results indicate that for small values of k, the cube root is a more effective normalizing transformation than the square root, although either one would probably suffice for practical purposes.

implies that all the remaining observations follow a specified probability distribution, while the outliers come from distributions of that form (perhaps) but with different parameters. Thus, we may suppose that almost all the observations conform to a multivariate normal distribution with mean $\boldsymbol{\mu}^T = (\mu_1,\mu_2, \ldots ,\mu_k)$ and variance-covariance matrix $\boldsymbol{\Sigma}$, but that possibly one or a very few (say, s) of the n observed vectors are affected by systematic biases that change their mean values to $\boldsymbol{\mu} + \mathbf{a}_1$, $\boldsymbol{\mu} + \mathbf{a}_2, \ldots , \boldsymbol{\mu} + \mathbf{a}_s$, respectively. Notice that both the $\boldsymbol{\mu}$'s and the $\mathbf{a}$'s are k-dimensional vectors. Another alternative would be that no systematic biases exist, but that some rare random circumstance has increased the standard deviation of each variable by a constant percentage. The methods described below are valid regardless of which explanation is correct.

Multivariate outliers are often difficult to detect simply as observations because, unlike univariate outliers, they will seldom appear clearly separate from the rest of the sample. For example, they might differ substantially from their fellows with respect to only one or two variables, or they might be only mildly different in all dimensions. However, in bivariate data with a high correlation, outliers may become evident when the paired variables are plotted against each other in a scatter diagram. This possibility may be exploited in multivariate data by selecting pairs of variables whose values are expected to correlate fairly closely. Biochemical test batteries often lend themselves to such pairing off. In general, however, we need to reduce multivariate data to a univariate index whose values can then be sorted and any outliers detected. Healy's idea (1968) of plotting the cube root (or square root) of the estimated quadratic form $\hat{Q}_k$ on normal probability paper serves to isolate outliers as well as to test the normality of the remaining observation vectors. He suggested, therefore, that individual values of $\sqrt{\hat{Q}_k}$ or $\sqrt[3]{\hat{Q}_k}$ be replotted on normal probability paper after deleting the apparent outliers and recomputing the mean vector and variance-covariance matrix

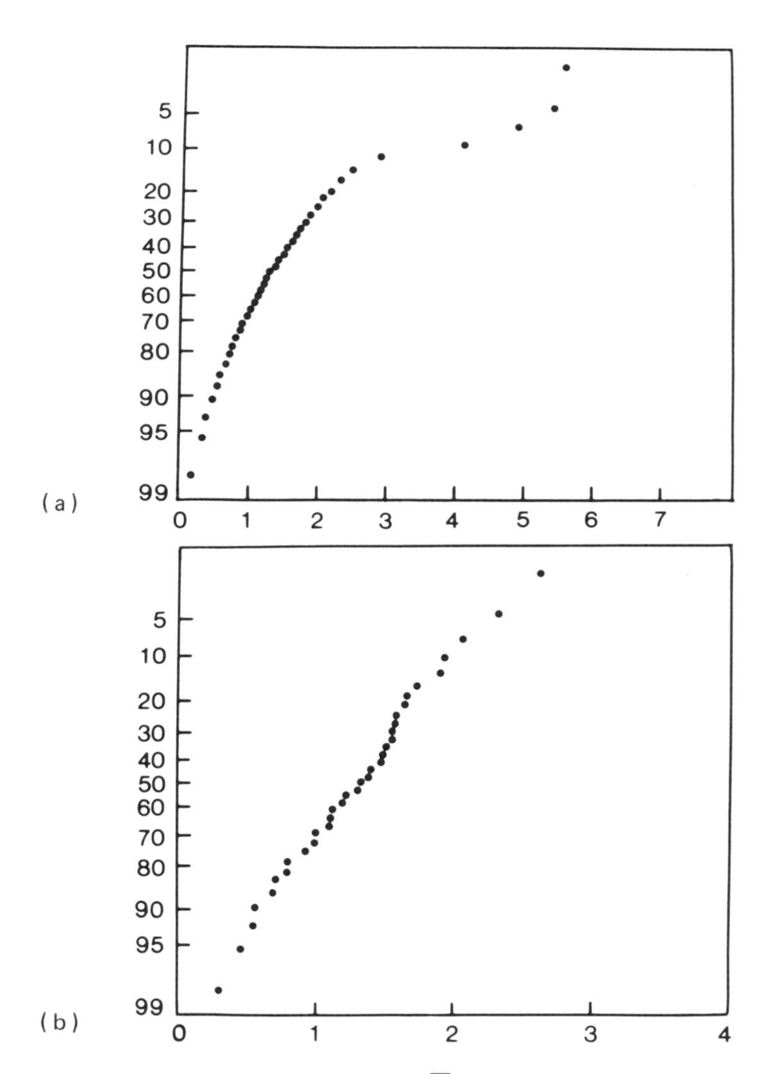

FIGURE 2.4 Normal plots of $\sqrt{\hat{Q}_2}$ for the distribution of log daily fat intake and log serum cholesterol in a sample of 39 hospital patients. (a) Complete sample. (b) Omitting 4 extreme values (Healy, 1968).

from the remaining data. If these new values of $\hat{Q}_k$ plot approximately linearly, the reduced database conforms to multivariate normality. To illustrate, Figure 2.4, taken from Healy's paper, shows plots of $\sqrt{\hat{Q}_2}$ before and after omitting four extreme values in a study of log daily fat intake and log serum cholesterol in 39 hospital patients.

More formal statistical methods for detecting outliers are discussed by Barnett and Lewis (1978). The basic index variable is the ratio of two determinants, say $\lambda(j) = |\mathbf{A}^{(j)}|/|\mathbf{A}|$, where $\mathbf{A}$ is the matrix of sums of squares and crossproducts of all observations about the vector of observed means, i.e.,

$$\mathbf{A} = \sum_{i=1}^{n} (\mathbf{x}_i - \mathbf{m})(\mathbf{x}_i - \mathbf{m})^T$$

and $\mathbf{A}^{(j)}$ is the same matrix with the jth observation vector deleted ($j = 1, \ldots, n$). The test statistic r_1 is the minimum of the n computed values of $\lambda(j)$ since the deleted observation in r_1 will be the farthest from the mean vector. Barnett and Lewis show that minimizing $\lambda(j)$ is equivalent to maximizing the quadratic form used by Healy, namely

$$\hat{Q}_{kj} = (\mathbf{x}_j - \mathbf{m})^T\mathbf{S}^{-1}(\mathbf{x}_j - \mathbf{m})$$

where $\mathbf{m}$ and $\mathbf{S}$ are the sample estimates of the mean vector and variance-covariance matrix. Their book includes a table of the 5% and 1% significance levels for testing the maximum value of $\hat{Q}_{kj}$. Reproduced here in Table 2.1, these percentage points provide a way of testing whether the largest value in a Healy plot represents a "significant" outlier.

Barnett and Lewis's table was abstracted from a comprehensive work by Wilks (1963) who also derived statistical tests for assessing the significance of pairs, triples, and quadruples of outliers (i.e., $s = 2$, 3, or 4). This involves computing ratios $\lambda(j_1, \ldots, j_s)$, where the numerator is the determinant

TABLE 2.1 Critical Values for 5% and 1% Tests of Discordancy of a Single Outlier in a k-multivariate Normal Sample of Size n

Sample size (n)	Number of variables (k)							
	$k = 2$		$k = 3$		$k = 4$		$k = 5$	
	5%	1%	5%	1%	5%	1%	5%	1%
5	3.17	3.19						
6	4.00	4.11	4.14	4.16				
7	4.71	4.95	5.01	5.10	5.12	5.14		
8	5.32	5.70	5.77	5.97	6.01	6.09	6.11	6.12
9	5.85	6.37	6.43	6.76	6.80	6.97	7.01	7.08
10	6.32	6.97	7.01	7.47	7.50	7.79	7.82	7.98
12	7.10	8.00	7.99	8.70	8.67	9.20	9.19	9.57
14	7.74	8.84	8.78	9.71	9.61	10.37	10.29	10.90
16	8.27	9.54	9.44	10.56	10.39	11.36	11.20	12.02
18	8.73	10.15	10.00	11.28	11.06	12.20	11.96	12.98
20	9.13	10.67	10.49	11.91	11.63	12.93	12.62	13.81
25	9.94	11.73	11.48	13.18	12.78	14.40	13.94	15.47
30	10.58	12.54	12.24	14.14	13.67	15.51	14.95	16.73
35	11.10	13.20	12.85	14.92	14.37	16.40	15.75	17.73
40	11.53	13.74	13.36	15.56	14.96	17.13	16.41	18.55
45	11.90	14.20	13.80	16.10	15.46	17.74	16.97	19.24
50	12.23	14.60	14.18	16.56	15.89	18.27	17.45	19.83
100	14.22	16.95	16.45	19.26	18.43	21.30	20.26	23.17
200	15.99	18.94	18.42	21.47	20.59	23.72	22.59	25.82
500	18.12	21.22	20.75	23.95	23.06	26.37	25.21	28.62

Source: Barnett and Lewis (1978).

of the matrix **A** with s observation vectors deleted. The test statistic r_s is the square root of the minimum value of $\lambda(j_1, \ldots, j_s)$. The Barnett and Lewis book also includes a table of 5% and 1% significance values of r_2 for $k = 2$ to 5 and a wide range of values of n. However, when n is large, the number of real outliers may easily exceed two to four, so that a graphical method like Healy's would be necessary to find and, at least indirectly, test them. Barnett and Lewis discuss briefly other graphical procedures for detecting multivariate outliers, such as principal component analysis and the use of various distance functions.

2.6 USE OF TRANSFORMATIONS TO IMPROVE NORMALITY

Even when no significant outliers appear, or they have all been removed from the database, a Healy plot of the remaining data may show curvature, a sign of nonnormality. With clinical laboratory data, the curve is likely to be concave, the result of positive skewness in the distributions of some variables. Probably the most effective way in practice to improve multivariate normality is to examine the distribution of each variable separately, for example, by plotting reference values on normal probability paper and computing coefficients of skewness and kurtosis. It is well known that such transforming functions as the logarithm or square root may substantially reduce positive skewness. Figure 2.5(a) and (b) shows plots of reference values for serum haptoglobin in mg/100 ml (as hemoglobin binding capacity) published by Reed et al. (1971) on the original scale and after transformation to square roots. Coefficients of skewness and kurtosis are given.

The general power transform $z = x^\lambda$ $(\lambda \neq 0)$ has been discussed in the statistical literature going back to the early 1940s. Its use was especially stimulated by the work of Box and Cox (1964), modifying and generalizing an earlier landmark study of transformations by Tukey (1957). The simple power transform examined by Box and Cox was

$$z = \begin{cases} (x^\lambda - 1)/\lambda & (\lambda \neq 0) \\ \log x & (\lambda = 0) \end{cases}$$

($\lambda = \frac{1}{2}$ represents the square root transform.)

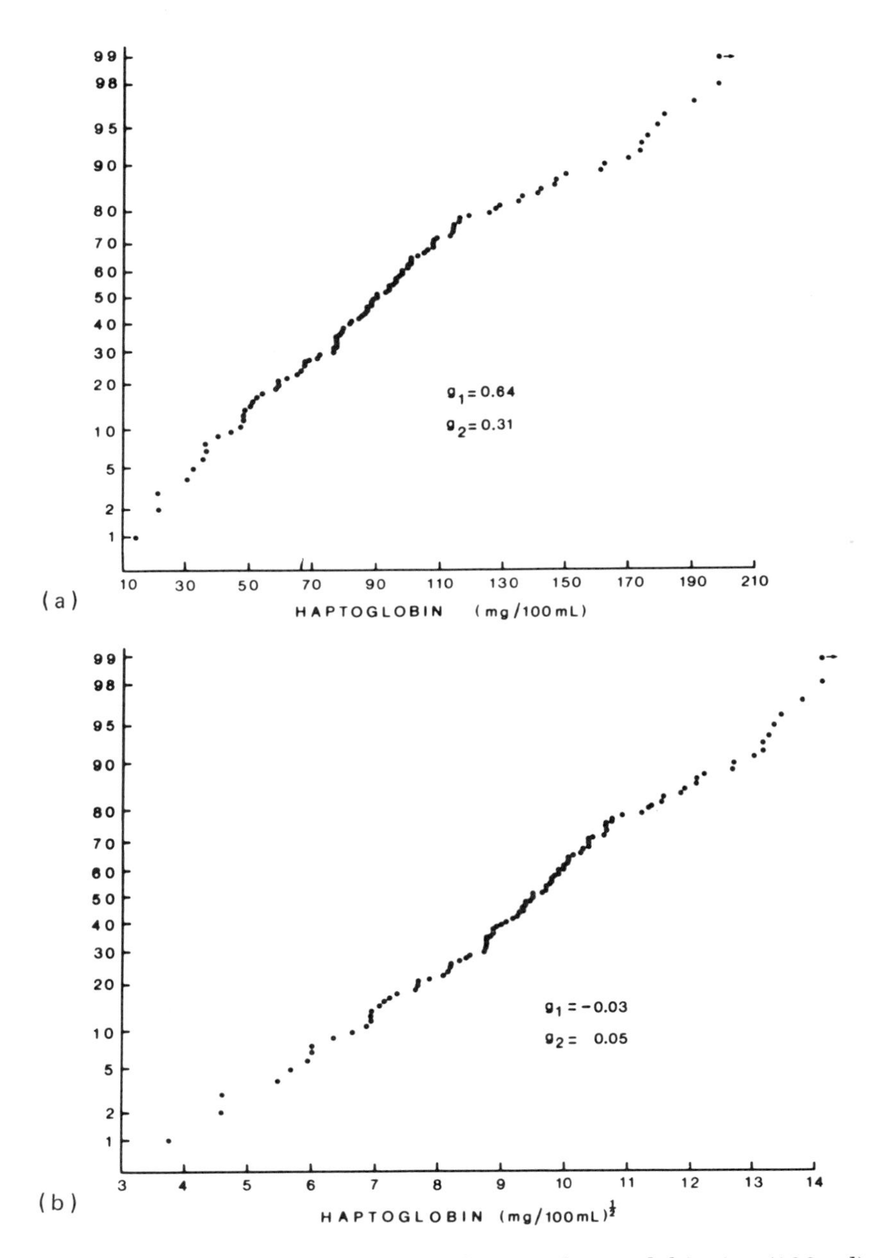

FIGURE 2.5 (a) Probability plot of serum haptoglobin (mg/100 ml) on original scale. (b) After square root transform. (Data from Reed, Henry, and Mason, 1981.)

The maximum likelihood estimate of λ must be obtained iteratively. Usually, however, the likelihood curve around the maximum is not sharply peaked, so that a convenient fraction close to the peak value may be chosen for λ.

Working with biochemical data, Harris and DeMets (1972), and Flynn et al. (1974) showed that the extended log transform, $\log(x + C)$, where C is a constant such that $(x + C) > 0$ for all values of X can sometimes be an improvement over $\log x$ alone. An initial estimate of C may be derived from a formula given by Johnson (1949), which involves solving a cubic equation. The final choice of C must be determined iteratively by trial and error.

The power and log transforms are intended primarily to remove skewness, either to the left or right. Various workers in clinical chemistry (Harris and DeMets, 1972; Boyd and Lacher, 1982; Solberg, 1983) have found that at times some degree of kurtosis remains after applying these transforms. To remove positive residual kurtosis (long tails on both sides), Harris and DeMets (1972), citing theory originally developed by Johnson (1949), suggested the inverse hyperbolic sine, $y = \log\{z + (z^2 + 1)^{1/2}\}$, as a second-stage transform after eliminating skewness; z should first be standardized by subtracting its mean and dividing by its standard deviation. Boyd and Lacher (1982) found the direct hyperbolic sine, $y = (e^z - e^{-z})/2$, useful in removing negative residual kurtosis (nonnormal peakedness).

Normalizing transforms often have the additional benefit of producing a new variable whose standard deviation is relatively constant, independent of the mean value of the measurement. Thus, a constant coefficient of variation, implying a standard deviation proportional to the mean (often seen in enzyme measurements, for example) leads to positive skewness correctable by a log transform which also stabilizes the standard deviation. Normalization of the individual variables in a multivariate set may, of course, require different transforming functions. The improvement in overall multivariate normality will most easily be indicated by a posttransform Healy plot.

APPENDIX

The "expected" or mean value of a random variable X, written $E(X)$, is defined for a continuous variable by the formula, $E(X) = \int_R x\ \mathrm{pr}(x)\, dx$, where $\int_R$ signifies integration over the entire range of X. For a normally distributed variable

$$
\begin{aligned}
E(X) &= (2\pi\sigma^2)^{-1/2} \int_{-\infty}^{\infty} x \exp[(-2\sigma^2)^{-1}(x - \mu)^2]\, dx \\
&= (2\pi)^{-1/2} \int_{-\infty}^{\infty} (\mu + \sigma z) \exp(-z^2/2)\, dz \\
&\quad \text{where } z = (x - \mu)/\sigma \\
&= \mu \int_{-\infty}^{\infty} (2\pi)^{-1/2} \exp(-z^2/2)\, dz \\
&\quad + \sigma \int_{-\infty}^{\infty} z(2\pi)^{-1/2} \exp(-z^2/2)\, dz \\
&= \mu
\end{aligned}
$$

since the first integral term equals unity while the second is zero.

The variance of a random variable X is defined in statistical theory as the expected value of the squared deviation of a value from its mean; that is,

$$
\begin{aligned}
\mathrm{Var}\,(X) &= E(X - EX)^2 \qquad \text{which for a continuous variable} \\
&= \int_R (x - EX)^2\, \mathrm{pr}(x)\, dx
\end{aligned}
$$

When X is normally distributed,

$$
\begin{aligned}
\mathrm{Var}\,(X) &= \int_{-\infty}^{\infty} (x-\mu)^2 (2\pi\sigma^2)^{-1/2} \exp[(-2\sigma^2)^{-1}(x-\mu)^2]\, dx \\
&= \int_{-\infty}^{\infty} x^2 (2\pi\sigma^2)^{-1/2} \exp[(-2\sigma^2)^{-1}(x-\mu)^2]\, dx - \mu^2
\end{aligned}
$$

$$= \mu^2 \int_{-\infty}^{\infty} (2\pi)^{-1/2} \exp(-z^2/2)\, dz + 2\mu\sigma \int_{-\infty}^{\infty} z(2\pi)^{-1/2}$$

$$\exp(-z^2/2)dz + \sigma^2 \int_{-\infty}^{\infty} z^2 (2\pi)^{-1/2} \exp(-z^2/2)\, dz - \mu^2 = \sigma^2$$

since the first and third integrals are unity, and the second zero.

Thus, the parameters of the normal distribution are its mean (μ) and variance (σ^2), respectively.

REFERENCES

Anderson, T. W. (1958). *An Introduction to Multivariate Statistical Analysis*. Wiley, New York.

Barnett, V., and Lewis, T. (1978). Outliers in statistical data. In *Outliers in Multivariate Data*. Wiley, New York, Chapter 6.

Box, G. E. P., and Cox, D. R. (1964). An analysis of transformations. *J. Roy. Stat. Soc., Ser. B 26*, 211–252.

Boyd, J. C., and Lacher, D. A. (1982). A multi-stage Gaussian transformation algorithm for clinical laboratory data. *Clin. Chem. 28*, 1735–1741.

Dixon, W. J., and Massey, F. J. (1969). *Introduction to Statistical Analysis*. McGraw-Hill, New York.

Flynn, F. V., Piper, K. A. J., Garcia-Webb, P., McPherson, K., and Healy, M. J. R. (1974). The frequency distributions of commonly determined blood constituents in healthy blood donors. *Clin. Chim. Acta 52*, 163–171.

Harris, E. K., and DeMets, D. L. (1972). Estimation of normal ranges and cumulative proportions by transforming observed distributions to Gaussian form. *Clin. Chem. 18*, 605–612;

Healy, M. J. R. (1968). Multivariate normal plotting. *Appl. Stat. 17*, 157–161.

Johnson, N. L. (1949). Systems of frequency curves generated by methods of translation. *Biometrika 36*, 149–176.

Johnson, N. L., and Kotz, S. (1972). Bivariate and trivariate normal distributions. In *Distributions in Statistics: Continuous Multivariate Distributions*. Wiley, New York, Chapter 36, p. 88.

Mood, A. M. (1950). *Introduction to the Theory of Statistics*. McGraw-Hill, New York.

Morrison, D. F. (1976). The multivariate normal distribution. In *Multivariate Statistical Methods*. McGraw-Hill, Kogakusha, Tokyo.

Reed, A. H., Henry, R. J., and Mason, W. B. (1971). Influence of statistical method used on the resulting estimate of normal range. *Clin. Chem. 17*, 275–284.

Solberg, H. E. (1983). *REFVAL—Technical Report*. Rikshospitalet, Oslo, Norway.

Tukey, J. W. (1957). On the comparative anatomy of transformations. *Ann. Math. Statist. 28*, 602–632.

Wilks, S. S. (1963). Multivariate statistical outliers. *Sankhyā, A25*, 407–426.

3

The Multivariate Reference Region and Other Tools for Interpreting Multivariate Profiles

3.1
INTRODUCTION

A single measurement of some biochemical quantity in a patient's blood or urine is of no value to the attending physician unless he or she can extract information from it about the patient's medical condition. This requires comparing the result to another number or range of numbers believed to represent the analyte's concentration in a given medical condition. For example, when the condition represented is that of a healthy individual, a "normal range" is commonly used for comparison. However, it is also possible, at least in principle, to obtain representative values from patients with specific diseases. Recognizing this, many clinical chemists today use the more general term "reference range."

It used to be that the quoted normal values were, in fact, the average and range observed in a small group of human volunteers, often laboratory workers or medical students. Following World War II, studies based on larger and less selective groups (e.g., Wootton et al., 1951) demonstrated that in apparently healthy persons, the measured values (or their logarithms) often appear to follow a normal distribution (hence the confusion between medically "normal" and statistically "normal"). The normal or reference range then came to be defined by limits that enclosed a specified proportion of the population, usually 95%. More recently, this definition of the univariate reference range has been extended to the multivariate reference region, defined mathematically in Chapter 2 for the multivariate normal distribution.

We should mention some statistical, and even practical, problems implied in the use of a population-based range. For example, what "population" is appropriate? Suppose the result requiring interpretation is a serum thyroxine (T-4) measurement in a 37-year-old woman at an outpatient clinic in Cleveland, Ohio. Should the physician compare this result with a reference range derived from all serum T-4 values observed in 35- to 40-year-old, nonthyroid-diseased women seen at this clinic since the present method of T-4 analysis was put into use? Perhaps this narrowly defined population of values is not immediately available, or the number of patients is too small. Is the doctor justified then in relying on a textbook range, based perhaps on an unquoted study of so-called healthy individuals, maybe classified by sex but not by age, from some far-off geographic location? Would the range supplied by the manufacturer of the analyzer be more suitable for comparison? Should each hospital or clinic laboratory maintain its own bank of patient data from which reference ranges may be computed for use by its clinical staff? The transferability of reference ranges is a large and important problem but beyond the scope of this book. We may note in passing that the most reliable reference value in the situation described above would probably be an earlier measurement of T-4 in the same patient, and, if such were available, the doctor would undoubtedly refer to it. In Chapter 8, we will discuss in detail some statistical methods to aid in interpreting serial values.

Before turning to the statistics of reference ranges and regions, several remarks are in order:

1. We shall consider only reference values from normally distributed variables. This is because for practical calculation and use we have to restrict discussion of reference regions to those obtained from multivariate normal distributions. Thus, we shall not review nonparametric reference ranges that make no assumption concerning the mathematical form of underlying distributions.

2. We shall speak of estimates of means, variances, and covariances from random samples of a population. Only rarely in clinical chemistry have truly random methods of selecting individuals been employed; in fact, the population the individuals are supposed to represent is often not clearly defined. For two notable exceptions, see Munan et al. (1978) and a report from the U.S. National Center for Health Statistics (1978). We have two excuses for appealing to random sampling theory in deriving reference regions: (a) statistically random

samples for determining reference values have been collected in the past and may be again sometime; and (b) error formulas based on random sample estimates adjust for sample size and thus distinguish between smaller and larger samples. Assuming large populations, such distinctions are worthwhile.

3. There are other sources of variation among values observed in different persons besides the genetic or long-term behavorial ones. In particular, adequate control should be exercised over conditions surrounding taking of the fluid specimen and preparation of the patient. These "pre-analytical" sources of variation have been discussed at length in a recent review by Statland and Winkel (1977). Finally, the Expert Panel on the Theory of Reference Values, appointed by the International Federation of Clinical Chemistry, is preparing a series of recommendations for selecting reference subjects, controlling pre-analytic as well as analytic sources of variation, and calculating (nonparametric) reference ranges as well as confidence limits for selected percentiles. Clearly, the clinical chemical profession has made much progress within the last decade alone towards developing a sound scientific basis for the production of reference values, with emphasis on univariate ranges.

3.2 UNIVARIATE REFERENCE RANGES

In this section, we want to review briefly the statistical theory underlying the use of univariate reference ranges in clinical chemistry. As mentioned above, the function of a reference range is to provide the chemist or physician with a guide for interpreting a measured value of some analyte in a given patient. The range is calculated from measurements of this analyte in people who represent a sample from some definable population, although we may know little about the characteristics of this population. Let us assume that the measured values (or some transformation of them) in all individuals of the population are distributed in a normal distribution—the familiar bell-shaped curve—with mean μ and standard deviation σ. Then $100(1 - \alpha)\%$ of these values will lie between the limits $\mu - |z(\alpha/2)|\sigma$ and $\mu + |z(\alpha/2)|\sigma$, where $z(\alpha/2)$ is called a standard normal deviate whose numerical value may be found in tables of areas under the normal curve. For example, when $\alpha = 0.05$, $|z(\alpha/2)| = 1.96$, and 95% of the values in the population lie between the limits $\mu \pm 1.96\sigma$. When $\alpha = 0.2$, $|z(\alpha/2)| = 1.28$, and the limits $\mu \pm 1.28\sigma$ enclose 80% of the values. But this is only theory, because we can almost never test every individual in the population, and, even if we could, our efforts would yield no more than a snapshot in time for each person. Measured six months or even one week later, that person would probably show a slightly different result.

Thus, the real population of reference values is infinite in size, and at best we can obtain a more or less random sample of size n, whose mean $\bar{x}$ and standard deviation s are estimates of the corresponding population parameters, μ and σ. Another random sample of the same size would probably produce somewhat different values of $\bar{x}$ and s. Therefore, we cannot be 100% sure that any finite interval $\bar{x} \pm |z(\alpha/2)| \cdot s$ will include $100(1 - \alpha)\%$ of the population. However, for any value of α and sample size n, we can determine a (positive) multiplier $c(\alpha,n,\gamma)$ that will provide 100γ percent *confidence* that the interval $\bar{x} \pm c(\alpha,n,\gamma) \cdot s$ includes at least $100(1 - \alpha)\%$ of all values in the underlying population. Such an interval is called a "tolerance interval," and its meaning is clearly more complicated than that of $\mu \pm 1.96\sigma$. The latter represents a limiting tolerance interval for $\alpha = 0.05$ and $\gamma = 1$ as n becomes larger and larger.

Tables of $c(\alpha,n,\gamma)$ may be found in various statistical texts (e.g., Documenta Geigy, 1970; and Dixon and Massey, 1969) for various combinations of α, n and γ, assuming a normally distributed population of values of the measured variable. Consider, for example, a random sample of 100 observations from a normal distribution, with sample mean $\bar{x}$ and standard deviation s. Setting $\alpha = 0.05$ and $\gamma = 0.95$, $c(.05,100,0.95) =$

2.233, about 14% larger than 1.96. That is, the interval $\bar{x} \pm 2.233s$ will cover 95% of the population in 95% of cases when the statistics $\bar{x}$ and s are derived from random samples of size 100. For samples of size 1000, the multiplier c is reduced to 2.036. On the other hand, if we wish to retain the commonly used multiplier of 2, a sample size of 650 would be required to maintain even 75% confidence that the interval $\bar{x} \pm 2s$ contains 95% of the population. That is, in only 75% of cases where $\bar{x}$ and s are computed from samples of size 650 would the interval $\bar{x} \pm 2s$ include 95% of the values in the population.

It would seem that the statistical tolerance interval is what clinical chemists have in mind when they speak of a reference range derived from a sample of individuals representing some defined population. Yet, while chemists or clinicians may think of a reference range as an interval very likely to include some high proportion of all the values in the population, they use reference ranges for a quite different purpose. This purpose is to predict the interval in which a single measured value of the analyte would lie if the patient being tested were, in fact, typical of the population from which the reference range was derived. A prediction reference interval for a single value must take into account not only variability in the mean and standard deviation of random samples but also the uncertainty of a single observation. The former source of variation would be accounted for if we multiplied the estimated standard error of the mean, $s/\sqrt{n}$, by Student's t for a given level of α and $(n - 1)$ degrees of freedom. The latter source would be recognized by multiplying s alone by Student's t. In fact, we add the two variance components s^2/n and s^2, then take the square root to obtain the reference predictive range,

$$\bar{x} \pm (1 + 1/n)^{1/2} t(^1/_2\alpha; n - 1) \cdot s \qquad (3.1)$$

Guttman (1970) has shown that this interval is equivalent to a tolerance interval for which $\gamma = 0.5$; that is, this interval has only a 50/50 chance of containing $100(1 - \alpha)\%$ of the values in the reference population. Another way of expressing the same idea (assuming a normal distribution) is to say that, on the average, this interval will include $100(1 - \alpha)\%$ of the reference population. It is therefore also called an expected $100(1 - \alpha)$ percent tolerance interval. Even for moderate sample sizes like $n = 100$, the width of the range $\bar{x} \pm (1 + 1/n)^{1/2}\, t(\frac{1}{2}\alpha; n - 1)\cdot s$ is not much greater than $\bar{x} \pm 2s$, the common univariate reference range. So, in a rather roundabout way, we have found statistical justification for the reference range clinical chemists and physicians have been using for many years: the mean plus and minus two standard deviations.

3.3 MULTIVARIATE REFERENCE REGIONS

In Chapter 2, we drew attention to the ellipse that a plane parallel to the bivariate (x,y) plane would define if it cut through a bivariate normal surface. The equation for this ellipse was expressed in equation (2.4). We mentioned that the left-hand side,

$$(1 - \rho^2)^{-1}\left\{\frac{(x - \mu_x)^2}{\sigma_x^2} + \frac{(y - \mu_y)^2}{\sigma_y^2} - \frac{2\rho(x - \mu_x)(y - \mu_y)}{\sigma_x\sigma_y}\right\}$$

a random variable in x and y, is called a "quadratic" form in two variables, denoted by Q_2. It is distributed in a chi-square (χ^2) distribution with 2 degrees of freedom. Therefore, if we set this quadratic form equal to or less than the $(100\,P)$th percentile of this chi-square distribution and graphed all the paired x,y-values that satisfy this inequality, we would obtain a dense region of points bounded by the ellipse $Q_2 = \chi^2(P;2)$. This region, centered around the mean (μ_x,μ_y), contains $(100\,P)$

TABLE 3.1 (100 P)th Percentile of the Chi-square Distribution on k Degrees of Freedom for Various P-values: $\chi^2(P;k)^a$

Degrees of freedom (k)	Proportion (P)				
	0.50	0.80	0.90	0.95	0.99
1	0.46	1.64	2.71	3.84	6.64
2	1.39	3.22	4.61	5.99	9.21
3	2.37	4.64	6.25	7.82	11.35
4	3.36	5.99	7.78	9.49	13.28
5	4.35	7.29	9.24	11.07	15.09
6	5.35	8.59	10.65	12.59	16.81
7	6.35	9.80	12.02	14.07	18.48
8	7.34	11.03	13.36	15.51	20.09
9	8.34	12.24	14.68	16.92	21.67
10	9.34	13.44	15.99	18.31	23.21
15	14.34	19.31	22.31	25.00	30.58
20	19.34	25.04	28.41	31.41	37.57

[a] A comprehensive table of chi-square percentiles can be found in many textbooks or in Biometrika Tables for Statisticians, Volume I (1970).

percent of all possible (x,y) pairs constituting the bivariate normal distribution, equation (2.3). Thus, it represents the two-variable counterpart of the line between the points $\mu_x \pm |z(\alpha/2)|\sigma_x$, which contains $100\,P = 100(1 - \alpha)\%$ of the values of X constituting a univariate normal distribution. Incidentally, this elliptical region has the property of being the smallest area containing $(100\,P)\%$ of the paired values in the corresponding bivariate normal. To give some specific examples, using a table of percentiles of the chi-square distribution (Table 3.1), $Q_2 = 5.99$ defines an ellipse containing 95% of the (x,y)-values in a bivariate normal distribution. The ellipse $Q_2 = 3.22$ contains 80% of such pairs.

As stated in Chapter 2, the k-variate quadratic form (2.7) $Q_k = (\mathbf{x} - \boldsymbol{\mu})^T\boldsymbol{\Sigma}^{-1}(\mathbf{x} - \boldsymbol{\mu})$ is distributed as chi-square with k degrees of freedom. Thus, $Q_k = \chi^2(P;k)$ defines a hyperellipsoidal region in k-dimensional space containing $(100\,P)$

percent of all observation vectors in a k-variate normal distribution. Such regions qualify as multivariate reference regions when the parameters of the distribution (means, variances, and covariances) are known. But in the practical situation, these parameters are unknown and can only be estimated from a sample of individuals that we hope is representative of the desired population.*

By the same reasoning followed earlier with respect to univariate reference intervals, we are led to consider a k-variate predictive region as the reference region most useful to clinicians interested in the "typicality" of an observed set of test results. In a key paper on the subject of confidence, tolerance, and prediction regions for the multivariate normal distribution, Chew (1966) refers to a (100 P)% prediction region for a single observation vector in exactly the same way as does Guttman with respect to a single univariate result, namely, as a tolerance region which will, on the average, contain exactly (100 P)% of the population. Chew cites the following equation (Fraser and Guttman, 1956) for a (100 P)% prediction region, generalizing the bivariate ellipse to three or more dimensions:

$$(\mathbf{x} - \overline{\mathbf{x}})^T \mathbf{S}^{-1} (\mathbf{x} - \overline{\mathbf{x}}) = \frac{k(n^2 - 1)F(P;k,n - k)}{n(n - k)} \qquad (3.2)$$

where the left-hand side is the generalized quadratic form in standard matrix notation with $\mathbf{x}$ representing a vector of observations on k variables, $\overline{\mathbf{x}}$ the vector of observed means of the variables, and $\mathbf{S}$, the matrix of variances and covariances computed from the same sample of n observation vectors. On the right-hand side, $F(P;k,n - k)$ denotes the (100 P)th percentile of the F distribution for k and $n - k$ degrees of

*For example, a trivariate reference region for thyroid function tests in middle-aged women, based on data from 3777 healthy subjects, has been published by Kågedal et al. (1978). The boundary of the ellipsoidal region was set equal to the 95th percentile of the distribution of observed Q_3-values (8.49), rather than the corresponding chi-square value [$\chi^2(0.95;3)$] of 7.88.

TABLE 3.2 (100 P)th Percentile of the F Distribution for k and $n - k$ Degrees of Freedom $F(P;k,n - k)$[a] for $P = 0.95$

Value for $n - k$	Value for k									
	1	2	3	4	5	6	7	8	9	10
10	4.96	4.10	3.71	3.48	3.33	3.22	3.14	3.07	3.02	2.98
20	4.35	3.49	3.10	2.87	2.71	2.60	2.51	2.45	2.39	2.35
30	4.17	3.32	2.92	2.69	2.53	2.42	2.33	2.27	2.21	2.16
40	4.08	3.23	2.84	2.61	2.45	2.34	2.25	2.18	2.12	2.08
50	4.03	3.18	2.79	2.56	2.40	2.29	2.20	2.13	2.07	2.03
60	4.00	3.15	2.76	2.53	2.37	2.25	2.17	2.10	2.04	1.99
70	3.98	3.13	2.74	2.50	2.35	2.23	2.14	2.07	2.02	1.97
80	3.96	3.11	2.72	2.49	2.33	2.21	2.13	2.06	2.00	1.95
90	3.95	3.10	2.71	2.47	2.32	2.20	2.11	2.04	1.99	1.94
100	3.94	3.09	2.70	2.46	2.31	2.19	2.10	2.03	1.97	1.93
200	3.89	3.04	2.65	2.42	2.26	2.14	2.06	1.98	1.93	1.88
300	3.87	3.03	2.63	2.40	2.24	2.13	2.04	1.97	1.91	1.86
500	3.86	3.01	2.62	2.39	2.23	2.12	2.03	1.96	1.90	1.85
1000	3.85	3.00	2.61	2.38	2.22	2.11	2.02	1.95	1.89	1.84

[a]A comprehensive table of F-distribution percentiles can be found in many textbooks or in Biometrika Tables for Statisticians, Volume I (1970).

freedom. We would conventionally take $P = 0.95$ (see Table 3.2). For reasonably large n, we can, of course, replace $(n^2 - 1)/n$ by n on the right-hand side.

How would we use equation (3.2) to judge whether an observed vector or "profile" of, say, 3 biochemical test values in a patient fell within a 95% predictive reference region for the variables? Suppose the region had been computed from a cross-sectional study of 100 healthy persons, i.e., 100 trivariate sets of observations, one set per person. Assuming that these data followed a trivariate normal distribution, perhaps requiring transformation of one or more of the variables to another measurement scale, they would be fully characterized by a profile of mean values $\bar{\mathbf{x}}$ and a variance-covariance matrix $\mathbf{S}$. Then, calling the newly observed profile $\mathbf{x}_0$, we would compute $(\mathbf{x}_0 - \overline{\mathbf{x}})^T\mathbf{S}^{-1}(\mathbf{x}_0 - \overline{\mathbf{x}})$. If this result exceeded (3 × 100/97) times 2.70, the upper 5% significance level of the F distribution with 3 and 97 degrees of freedom, we would conclude that the observed profile lay outside the reference region, indicating that the patient was "significantly" different from the reference population. Note that the criterion used here, 2.70 (300/97) = 8.34, is slightly more "conservative" than the chi-square value $[\chi^2(0.95;3) = 7.88]$ which would have been our criterion if we had known the values of the parameters in the quadratic form [equation (2.7)].

We shall meet this criterion again in Chapter 8 on time series analysis. There we use the F-distribution to calculate a forecast range for the t-th profile in a series, given a set of $(t - 1)$ mutually independent preceding profiles. In this case, $n = t - 1$, often less than 10, and use of the large-sample chi-square approximation rather than the exact F-criterion would be grossly misleading.

When the observed profile $\mathbf{x}_0$ is substituted for the vector $\mathbf{x}$ in the quadratic form on the left-hand side of equation (3.2), the result is known as the "generalized" distance D^2 (Mahalanobis, 1936) between $\mathbf{x}_0$ and the mean of the reference population, i.e., $D^2(\mathbf{x}_0) = (\mathbf{x}_0 - \overline{\mathbf{x}})^T\mathbf{S}^{-1}(\mathbf{x}_0 - \overline{\mathbf{x}})$. When $D^2(\mathbf{x}_0) \leq C$, where C represents the right side of equation (3.2), the profile is inside the reference region; otherwise, it is outside. Calculating and interpreting $D^2(\mathbf{x}_0)$ for $k \geq 3$ generally requires a fully automated (computerized) procedure.

Example

The data in Table 3.3 refer to a profile of three classical laboratory tests (urea, uric acid, creatinine) that were measured in a reference sample of 284 healthy individuals (Albert, 1981). It is seen that the tests are positively correlated, suggesting a multivariate interpretation of the results.

Consider now the following observed profile $\mathbf{x}_0$: urea = 5.4 mmol/L, uric acid = 298 μmol/L and creatinine = 78 μmol/L. Its distance to the estimated mean vector $\overline{\mathbf{x}}$ of the reference population equals

$$D^2(\mathbf{x}_0) = (\mathbf{x}_0 - \bar{\mathbf{x}})^T \mathbf{S}^{-1}(\mathbf{x}_0 - \bar{\mathbf{x}}) = 0.58$$

Calculating the right-hand side of equation (3.2), with $k = 3$, $n = 284$, and $F(0.95;3,281) = 2.64$, we obtain a critical value $C = 7.99$. Clearly, the observed profile is well within the 0.95 reference region, since $D^2(\mathbf{x}_0) < 7.99$. Conversely, the profile: urea = 6.6 mmol/L, uric acid = 387 μmol/L, creatinine = 62 μmol/L, yields a distance $D^2(\mathbf{x}_0) = 14.53$, much higher than 7.99. This profile should be considered highly abnormal from a multivariate standpoint.

The univariate 95% prediction reference intervals (equation 3.1) corresponding to these laboratory tests are, respectively,

urea:	2.9 − 7.3 mmol/L	$(5.1 \pm 1.00 \times 1.97 \times 1.1)$
uric acid:	183 − 423 μmol/L	$(303 \pm 1.00 \times 1.97 \times 61)$
creatinine:	57 − 113 μmol/L	$(85 \pm 1.00 \times 1.97 \times 14)$

since $(1 + 1/n)^{1/2} \simeq 1.00$ and $t(0.975;283) \simeq 1.97$. If these separate univariate ranges were used, the two observed profiles might escape notice since all results fall inside their own limits. In proceeding this way, we are actually defining a new reference region R' different from the ellipsoidal shaped region

TABLE 3.3 Mean Values, Standard Deviations, Covariances, and Correlations of Serum Urea (mmol/L), Uric Acid (μmol/L), and Creatinine (μmol/L) in a Random Sample of 284 Healthy Individuals

			Covariances and correlations[a]		
Analyte	Mean	(SD)	Urea	Uric acid	Creatinine
Urea	5.1	(1.1)	1.14	<u>0.23</u>	<u>0.39</u>
Uric acid	303	(61)	14.93	3724.3	<u>0.54</u>
Creatinine	85	(14)	6.02	473.3	205.5

[a]Correlations are underscored.
Source: Albert (1981).

R (3.2). This new region in three-dimensional space is a rectangular box whose sides are of lengths 4.4 (urea), 240 (uric acid), and 56 (creatinine). It contains approximately $100(0.95)^3\%$, or 86% of the reference population, because the three analytes are treated as if they were entirely independent of each other.

Multiple Univariate Reference Intervals

In general, for a k-dimensional profile, the region R' defined by the "multiple univariate" reference intervals covers a proportion $\beta = (0.95)^k$ of the reference population, a proportion rapidly diminishing with k. Alternatively, the probability of finding at least one result outside the reference interval increases with the number of tests measured. Therefore, using R' as if it were a 95% multivariate reference region would produce more than the expected number of false positives even if the tests were really uncorrelated. It is especially to avoid fruitless follow-up of sporadic univariate false positive results that multivariate reference regions have been recommended (Grams et al., 1972; and Winkel et al., 1972) when batteries of biochemical tests are routinely undertaken in patients of uncertain diagnosis. For example, computer-based simulation studies (Harris, 1981) have shown that when groups of three to five concurrent tests are run and only one test lies outside its 95% reference interval, causing the entire multivariate vector $\mathbf{x}_0$ to fall outside R', that vector has at least a 70% chance of lying inside the ellipsoidal reference region R. This probability increases with increasing correlation among test results, and would be over 85% for all batteries with more than five tests. Such results have also been verified in studies of real biochemical data obtained from apparently healthy persons undergoing periodic monitoring (Harris et al., 1982). A similar study of thyroid tests in patients has been reported by Kågedal et al. (1982).

We should note two caveats to the essentially sound recommendation that ellipsoidal multivariate predictive reference regions be computed and used in preference to separate univariate intervals. First, it is possible that the patient is suffering from a disease for which only one or two of a large battery of tests is truly diagnostic. In such a case, the other tests are only adding "noise," diverting attention, or, by use of a multivariate reference region based on all the tests, actually obscuring the important diagnostic signal. Thus, the clinical chemist or clinician should never ignore individual test results regardless of the statistical "significance," or lack thereof, of the multivariate profile. Second, there is a small but still finite probability, 0.015 or less, that a profile whose components all fell within their respective univariate intervals would lie outside the multivariate reference region R. The second profile example mentioned above illustrates this unusual situation. Later in this chapter, we shall refer again to this observed pattern and explain why it was indeed abnormal. Nevertheless, univariate reference ranges should always be available to consider when statistically significant multivariate profiles are being interpreted clinically.

With respect to laboratory computer operations and communication of results, the multivariate reference region raises some special problems, or better, challenges. The number of parameters (or their estimated values) that must be stored within the computer in order to develop a k-test region is equal to $k(k + 3)/2$. This includes the k test means and the $k(k + 1)/2$ elements of the covariance matrix (k variances, $k(k - 1)/2$ covariances) or of its inverse. For example, when $k = 3$, nine parameters must be estimated and stored. Finally, when k exceeds 3, there is no direct way to visualize the multivariate region. This may indicate that in practice multivariate profiles should include no more than three analytes. Perhaps larger test batteries should be subdivided into smaller groups of physiologically related tests.

Whether univariate or multivariate, the interpretation of observed results by means of the reference region is not an entirely satisfying procedure because it allows only a yes or no decision. A test result is "positive or abnormal" if it falls outside the reference region and "negative or normal" if it falls within. No account is made for the degree of positivity or negativity. Yet a person's state of health is a continuous variable; important differences may exist between the state indicated by a set of test values near the mean of the reference region and states represented by values just inside the boundary. Moreover, the boundary itself is derived from an arbitrary decision about what fraction of the population should be enclosed. The conventional 95% proportion originates from the 5% significance level commonly adopted in statistical practice.

Several methods have been proposed to counter these shortcomings of the reference region method. Each consists of transforming the observed profile into a univariate index such as a distance or a probability that locates the multivariate observation on a continuous scale with regard to the reference population. In the remaining portion of this chapter, we describe two of these procedures, first in the univariate case, then extended to higher dimensions. As usual, normality of the distributions is assumed.

3.4 THE *SD* UNIT

A. The Univariate Case

One of the simplest and most traditional methods for reporting analytical results consists of subtracting from the observed value x_0 the mean μ and by dividing by the standard deviation σ of the reference population.

$$z(x_0) = \frac{x_0 - \mu}{\sigma} \tag{3.3}$$

The dimensionless index $z(x_0)$ is called "the *SD* unit" associated with x_0 since it expresses the distance between the observation x_0 and the mean of the reference population in terms of the standard deviation (*SD*). The "*SD* unit system" was

TABLE 3.4 Application of the SD-unit System for Reporting and Interpreting Laboratory Results

Analyte	Observed result	Mean and SD of reference population		SD-unit[a]
	x_0	$\bar{x}$	s	$z(x_0) = (x_0 - \bar{x})/s$
Urea, mmol/L	6.6	5.1	1.1	+1.38
Uric acid, μmol/L	387	303	61	+1.38
Creatinine, μmol/L	62	85	14	−1.64

[a]The multivariate SD-unit for the observed profile is equal to 2.70.

initially proposed by Gullick and Schauble (1972). In practice, μ and σ are replaced by their usual estimates $\bar{x}$ and s, the sample mean and standard deviation, respectively.

The *SD* unit combines both sign and magnitude, indicating at once the direction and relative size of the difference between observed value and reference mean. The larger the numerical value of $z(x_0)$, the farther the observation from the reference population. Further, the index is dimensionless, making it possible to compare on a uniform scale results from different laboratory tests. For example, Table 3.4 shows the *SD* units for each of the tests in the "abnormal" renal profile given earlier. The creatinine result differs from the other two in two respects, as indicated by the values of $z(x_0)$. It is below the reference mean and, in terms of standard deviation, more distant from the reference population.

B. The Multivariate Extension

The concept of *SD* unit may be extended to the interpretation of observation vectors by using the generalized distance $D^2(\mathbf{x}_0)$ introduced earlier in the chapter. While this retains the idea of standardizing the difference between an observed profile and the population mean, the direction of the difference, represented by the sign of the *SD* unit, necessarily disappears since in higher dimensions the distance includes differences in either positive or negative directions.

We start with the multivariate distance,

$$D^2(\mathbf{x}_0) = (\mathbf{x}_0 - \overline{\mathbf{x}})^T\mathbf{S}^{-1}(\mathbf{x}_0 - \overline{\mathbf{x}})$$

Now suppose we divide $D^2(\mathbf{x}_0)$ by $C = k(n^2 - 1)\cdot F(0.95;k;n - k)/n(n- k)$, the boundary of the 95% predictive reference region [equation (3.2)]. Then, if the observed profile lies within (or on the boundary of) the reference region, $D^2(\mathbf{x}_0)/C \leq 1$. To complete the analogy with *SD* units, this ratio may be multiplied by $c^2 = (1 + 1/n)t^2(0.975;n - 1)$ or, for reference samples of $n \geq 100$, simply by $c^2 = 4$. Then, the final product,

$$Z(\mathbf{x}_0) = c[D^2(\mathbf{x}_0)/C]^{1/2} \qquad (3.4)$$

will exceed 2 when the observed profile lies outside the 95% reference region. More importantly, $Z(\mathbf{x}_0)$ becomes a continuous, easily recognized measure of the degree of dissimilarity between $\mathbf{x}_0$ and the reference population. When $k = 1$, $C = c^2$ and $Z(x_0) = z(x_0)$, the *SD* unit, thus making $Z(\mathbf{x}_0)$ a "multivariate *SD* unit," a direct extension of the univariate quantity.

As an example, consider again the profile in Table 3.4 for which we found earlier that $D^2(\mathbf{x}_0) = 14.53$ and $C = 7.99$, from which $Z(\mathbf{x}_0) = 2(14.53/7.99)^{1/2} = 2.70$, indicating strong disparity between the observation vector and the reference population. As mentioned earlier, this result is unusual in that the multivariate index is highly abnormal while all the separate chemistry values are within their respective univariate reference ranges. This paradox (Healy, 1969) becomes clearer when we recall that the multivariate *SD* index takes account of the correlations among laboratory tests, whereas the univariate *SD* units do not. We observe that the *SD* units associated with urea and uric acid have positive signs, but the deviation for creatinine is negative. This type of pattern would be quite unlikely in the reference population because the three constituents are positively correlated. Thus, while all results may be reasonably "normal" examined separately, they are highly "abnormal" as a multivariate profile.

The multivariate *SD* unit corresponding to an observed profile summarizes all the information contained in the profile with respect to the reference population. Its definition allows us to compare simultaneously profiles consisting of different numbers of tests. For example, a value of 3 has the same meaning whether derived from a single result, a 3-test profile, or a 20-test panel.

3.5 THE ATYPICALITY INDEX

This index (Albert, 1981) takes the *SD* unit a step further by determining the probability that the observed value x_0 or profile $\mathbf{x}_0$ belongs to the reference population (see Figure 3.1). In the univariate case, this probability would be derived from standard normal distribution tables for large reference samples ($n \geq 100$) or from tables of Student's t distribution for smaller samples.

The chief merit of the atypicality index lies in the fact that the idea may be extended straightforwardly (or at least by computer program) from the univariate to the multivariate case. Let

$$I(\mathbf{x}_0) = \mathrm{pr}[D^2(\mathbf{x}) \leq D^2(\mathbf{x}_0)] \tag{3.5}$$

where $D^2(\mathbf{x}_0) = (\mathbf{x}_0 - \boldsymbol{\mu})^T\boldsymbol{\Sigma}^{-1}(\mathbf{x}_0 - \boldsymbol{\mu})$. In practice, of course, $\boldsymbol{\mu}$ and $\boldsymbol{\Sigma}$ would be replaced by their estimates $\bar{\mathbf{x}}$ and $\mathbf{S}$, respectively. Then, $I(\mathbf{x}_0)$ may be estimated by the incomplete β-function, $\beta(U_0;k/2;(n - k)/2)$, where $U_0 = D^2(\mathbf{x}_0)/[D^2(\mathbf{x}_0) + (n^2 - 1)/n]$. An optimized algorithm for programming the computation of the incomplete β-function has been published

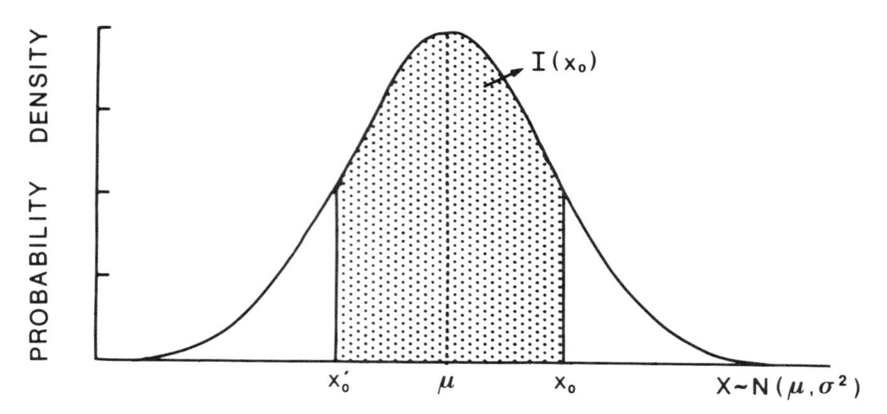

Figure 3.1: Atypicality index $I(x_0)$ associated with an observed laboratory value x_0. The point x_0 is the symmetric value of x_0 with respect to μ. (Adapted from Albert, 1981.)

(Majumber and Bhattacharjee, 1973). An excellent approximation to this function may also be obtained from normal distribution tables, as shown in the appendix to this chapter. When the ratio n/k is larger than 10, equation (3.5) can be calculated from the chi-square distribution on k degrees of freedom.

The multivariate atypicality index (3.5) represents the probability that the observed profile $\mathbf{x}_0$ departs from the reference population. It is therefore a dimensionless number ranging between zero and one. An index close to zero corresponds to a profile typical of the reference population, whereas an index close to one implies that the profile most likely arose from another population group. For example, an index value of 0.9 would indicate only a 10% chance that the observed profile came from the reference population of such profiles. The index provides the clinician with an easily interpretable measurement of how unusual the results might be relative to the reference population. This interpretation holds regardless of the number of variables included in the profile.

Example

Returning again to the profile in Table 3.4 with $D^2(\mathbf{x}_0) = 14.53$, and $(n^2 - 1)/n \simeq 284$, we calculate $U_0 = (14.53/298.53) = 0.0487$. Then, following the method outlined in the appendix, $w_1 = 1.89$, $w_2 = 0.7806$,

$$y = \frac{3[1.89(0.9992) - 0.7806(0.7778)]}{(0.0256 + 1.2187)^{1/2}} = 3.45$$

and $I(\mathbf{x}_0) \approx 1.00$, showing once more that this profile is very atypical of the reference population. Alternatively, since the ratio $n/k = 284/3$ is large, we can use a chi-square approximation on 3 degrees of freedom and find that $I(\mathbf{x}_0) = 0.9977$.

3.6 CONCLUDING REMARKS

Our emphasis in this chapter has been on multivariate reference methods for interpreting individual test profiles. Thus, we have proposed the prediction region as the most appropriate multivariate reference region. However, to overcome the disadvantage of any reference region, namely that it defines only two classes of results—"normal" or "abnormal"—we have also described two continuous indices: the *SD* unit, a relative distance, and the atypicality index, the probability of that distance. These measures allow a graded interpretation of just how unusual an observed profile is relative to its reference population. Both indices are applicable to univariate as well as multivariate test results, and the multivariate indices, whether in the form of a relative distance or its probability, are independent of the number of tests included in the profile. Such an index would seem to be particularly useful in either health screening or patient monitoring activities.

As noted above, a multivariate index can be compared with corresponding univariate indexes calculated separately for each constituent, but this may lead to opposite conclusions. In any specific decision-making process using laboratory test results, both forms can provide valuable information.

APPENDIX*

Normal approximation to the Incomplete β-function

The incomplete β-function, $\beta(U_0;\tfrac{1}{2}k;\tfrac{1}{2}(n - k))$ may be written

$$I(U_0) = \frac{1}{B(\frac{1}{2}k, \frac{1}{2}(n - k))} \int_0^{U_0} t^{(1/2k - 1)} (1 - t)^{1/2(n-k)-1} dt$$

where $0 \leq U_0 \leq 1$ is defined in the text, and $B(\quad)$ is a constant. Let $a = \tfrac{1}{2}k - 1$ and $b = \tfrac{1}{2}(n - k) - 1$. Then define a new variable y,

$$y = 3[w_1(1 - 1/9b) - w_2(1 - 1/9a)]/(w_1^2/b + w_2^2/a)^{1/2}$$
$$w_1 = (bU_0)^{1/3},\ w_2 = [a(1 - U_0)]^{1/3}$$

Then, $I(U_0) = (1/2\pi)^{1/2} \int_{-\infty}^{y} \exp(-z^2/2)\, dz$, the area under the standard normal curve from $-\infty$ to y.

REFERENCES

Albert, A. (1981). Atypicality indices as reference values for laboratory data. *Amer. J. Clin. Pathol. 76*, 421–425.

**Source*: *Handbook of Mathematical Functions* (1964).

Biometrika Tables for Statisticians, Volume I (1970). E. S. Pearson and H. O. Hartley (Eds.). Cambridge University Press, Cambridge, England.

Chew, V. (1966). Confidence, prediction and tolerance regions for the multivariate normal distribution. *J. Amer. Statist. Assoc. 61*, 605–617.

Dixon, W. J., and Massey, F. J., Jr. (1969). *Introduction to Statistical Analysis*, Table A-16, pp. 534–535. McGraw-Hill, New York.

Documenta Geigy Scientific Tables, Seventh Edition (1970). K. Diem and C. Lentner (Eds.). J. R. Geigy, S. A., Basel, Switzerland.

Fraser, D. A. S., and Guttman, I. (1956). Tolerance regions. *Annals of Math. Stat. 27*, 162–179.

Grams, R. R., Johnson, E. A., and Benson, E. S. (1972). Laboratory data analysis system: Section III—Multivariate normality. *Amer. J. Clin. Pathol. 58*, 188–200.

Gullick, H. D., and Schauble, M. K. (1972). SD unit system for standardized reporting and interpretation of laboratory data. *Amer. J. Clin. Pathol. 57*, 517–525.

Guttman, I. (1970). Statistical Tolerance Regions. Griffin, London.

Handbook of Mathematical Functions (1964). M. Abramowitz and I. A. Stegun (Eds.). U.S. Department of Commerce, National Bureau of Standards, Washington, D.C., Applied Mathematics Series, No. 55, 945 (26.5.21).

Harris, E. K. (1981). Statistical aspects of reference values in clinical pathology. In *Progress in Clinical Pathology, VIII*, M. Stefanini and E. Benson (Eds.). Grune and Stratton, New York, pp. 45–66.

Harris, E. K., Yasaka, T., Horton, M. R. and Shakarji, G. (1982). Comparing multivariate and univariate subject-specific reference regions for blood constituents in healthy persons. *Clinical Chemistry 28*, 422–426.

Healy, M. J. R. (1969). Rao's paradox concerning multivariate tests of significance. *Biometrics 25*, 411–413.

Kågedal, B., Larsson, L., Norr, A., and Toss, G. (1982). Trivariate evaluation of a thyroid hormone panel in clinical practice compared with multiple univariate evaluation. *Scand. J. Clin. Lab. Invest. 42*, 177–180.

Kågedal, B., Sandstrom, A., and Tibbling, G. (1978). Determination of a trivariate reference region for free thyroxine index, free triiodothyronine index, and thyrotropine from results obtained in a health survey of middle-aged women. *Clin. Chem. 24*, 1744–1750.

Mahalanobis, P. C. (1936). On the generalized distance in statistics. *Proc. Nat. Inst. Sci. (India) 12*, 49–55.

Majumber, K. L., and Bhattacharjee, G. P. (1973). The incomplete beta integral. *Applied Statist. 22*, 409–411.

Munan, L., Kelly, A., PetitClerc, C., and Billon, B. (1978). *Atlas of Blood Data.* University of Sherbrooke (Epidemiology Laboratory and Laboratory of Clinical Biochemistry, Faculty of Medicine), Sherbrooke, Quebec, Canada.

National Center for Health Statistics (1978). Total serum cholesterol levels of children 4–17 years, United States, 1971–74. *Vital and Health Statistics 11*, 207. Department of Health, Education, and Welfare, Washington, D.C., Pub. No. (PHS) 78-1655.

Statland, B. E., and Winkel, P. (1977). Effects of non-analytical factors on the intra- individual variation of analytes in the blood of healthy subjects: Consideration of preparation of the subject and time of venipuncture. *CRC Critical Reviews of Clinical Laboratory Science 8*, 105–144.

Winkel, P., Lyngbye, J., and Jorgensen, K. (1972). The normal region—A multivariate problem. *Scandin. J. Clin. Lab. Investig. 30*, 339–344.

Wootton, I. D. P., King, E. J., and Maclean Smith, J. (1951). The quantitative approach to hospital biochemistry: Normal values and the use of biochemical determinations for diagnosis and prognosis. *British Medical Bulletin 7*, 307–311.

4

Differential Diagnosis: Two Diagnostic Categories

4.1
INTRODUCTION

Reference regions are usually derived from samples of presumably healthy individuals. Therefore, referral of a laboratory result to such a region can indicate a general abnormality but is by itself useless for distinguishing among different disease conditions, i.e., for differential diagnosis. This task requires knowledge of the distribution of test values within each diagnostic category. In this chapter, we will discuss statistical methods for measuring the efficiency of laboratory tests and interpreting individual test results when distinguishing between two categories. For convenience, we will designate these categories as D and $\overline{D}$ and will assume that all individuals fall into either one or the other of these groups but not both. For example, D might be the class of diabetics, $\overline{D}$, all others, and the test, serum glucose, measured by a specific procedure. Figure 4.1 illustrates hypothetical distributions of test values in each of the two diagnostic classes. The point d on the scale of test values (x) represents a cutoff point such

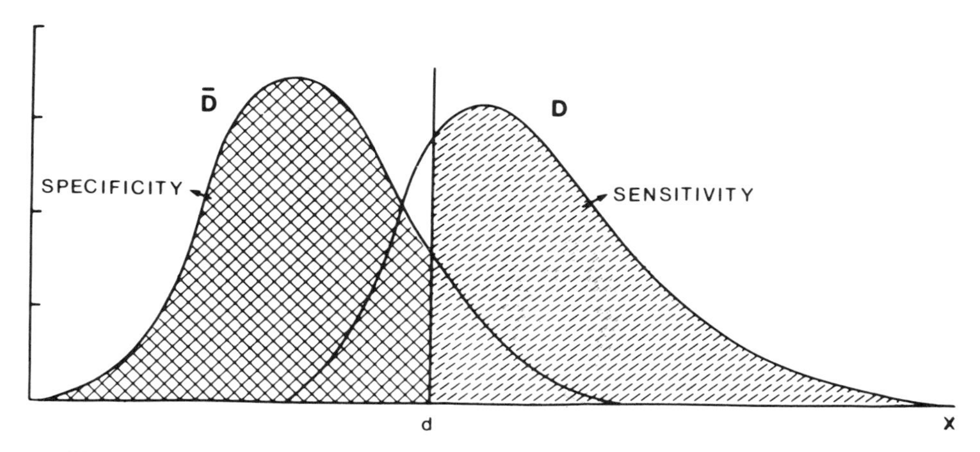

FIGURE 4.1 Overlapping distributions of a laboratory test X in two patient populations $\overline{D}$ and D. The value d defines a cutoff point on the x-scale.

that an observed value $x > d$ leads to the diagnosis D, while a value $x \leq d$ leads to the decision that $\overline{D}$ is the correct diagnostic class for this patient. Clearly, the smaller the overlap of the two distributions, the greater the probability that a correct decision will be made.

We want now to make a clear distinction between evaluation of the laboratory test (i.e., measuring its ability to separate the two populations D and $\overline{D}$) and interpretation of a particular test result (i.e., deciding whether the individual observed has come from Class D or Class $\overline{D}$). Of course, these concepts pertain to single tests as well as multivariate profiles, but different statistical indices are often used to deal with univariate and multivariate cases. Our chief aim in this chapter and the next will be to explore unifying techniques that may easily be generalized from one test to many.

4.2 SPECIFICITY AND SENSITIVITY

A single laboratory test is often evaluated in terms of its ability to distinguish between a healthy population $\overline{D}$ and a population of individuals suffering from a specified illness D. Although the test X may be a continuous variable, it is dichotomized by selecting a cutoff point d and defining a binary variable Y, such that

$$y = 0 \quad \text{when } x \leq d$$
$$y = 1 \quad \text{when } x > d$$

The specificity of a test is defined to be the proportion of healthy persons for which $y = 0$ (i.e., $x \leq d$). These are the "true negatives," and referring to Figure 4.1, their proportion is the area under the $\overline{D}$-distribution of X to the left of the ordinate at $x = d$. Conversely, the sensitivity of a test is defined to be the proportion of the diseased population for which $y =$

TABLE 4.1 Specificity and Sensitivity of a Laboratory Test X at Cutoff Point d

		Population	
		Healthy (D) ($\overline{D}$)	Diseased (D)
		Probabilities	
Laboratory test X	Negative $x \leqslant d$ $(y = 0)$	SP	1-SE
	Positive $x > d$ $(y = 1)$	1-SP	SE

[a]Or at least free of disease D.

1 (i.e., $x > d$). These are the "true positives," and their proportion is the area under the D-distribution to the right of the ordinate at $x = d$. Thus, in symbols,

$$\begin{aligned} \text{specificity} &= SP = \text{pr}(y = 0 | \overline{D}, d) \\ \text{sensitivity} &= SE = \text{pr}(y = 1 | D, d) \end{aligned} \tag{4.1}$$

These probabilities (Yerushalmy, 1947) and their complements are often displayed in a fourfold table, as in Table 4.1.

Notice that each column of Table 4.1 adds up to 1, but the rows do not. Since specificity and sensitivity depend on the choice of cutoff point d, we may express them as $SP = SP(d)$ and $SE = SE(d)$. Specificity and sensitivity vary inversely. Moving the cutoff point in Figure 4.1 from right to left decreases specificity while increasing sensitivity. At some point d^*, $SP(d^*) = SE(d^*) =$, say S^*, where $1/2 \leq S^* \leq 1$. A laboratory test for which $S^* = 1/2$ (perfect overlap) is useless for distinguishing the two diagnostic classes, whereas a test

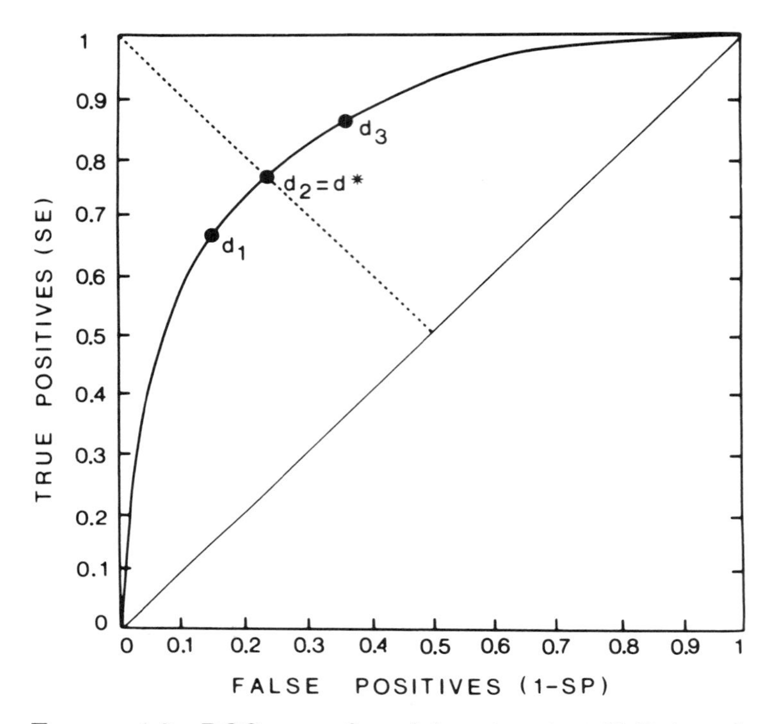

FIGURE 4.2 *ROC* curve for a laboratory test X. Points d_1, d_2, and d_3 on the curve represent strict, medium, and lenient decision criteria, respectively. The point d^* corresponds to equal sensitivity and specificity.

for which $S^* = 1$ is pathognomonic (complete separation). Note that the value of S^* does not depend on the decision point d, so that it can be used as a criterion for comparing the diagnostic efficiencies of different laboratory tests.

There is a classical graphic way of relating specificity and sensitivity to the point d, called the receiver operating characteristic (*ROC*) curve (Swets, 1979). As shown in Figure 4.2, the *ROC* curve is obtained by plotting the false positive rate $(1 - SP)$ versus the true positive rate (SE) for various values of d.

The value of S^* is obtained by intersecting the *ROC* curve with the dotted line $SE(d) = SP(d)$. A test is efficient if its

ROC curve concentrates in the upper left corner where both specificity and sensitivity are high. Conversely, an inefficient test would have a *ROC* curve close to the line $SE(d) = 1 - SP(d)$. Much recent work (McNeil and Hanley, 1984) has involved the area under the *ROC* curve, designated A_z and ranging in values from 0.5 (no apparent accuracy) to 1 (perfect accuracy). When estimating the areas A_z for two different laboratory tests by a maximum likelihood method rather than by eye, one also obtains their standard errors, thereby allowing for a statistical comparison of the two tests (Hanley and McNeil, 1983).

4.3 PREDICTIVE VALUE AND PRIOR PROBABILITY

We turn now to the question of interpreting the result of a dichotomized laboratory test in a given patient. The attending physician is interested in different probabilities than those defining specificity and sensitivity (equations 4.1). He or she is concerned chiefly with the probability that the patient being tested does indeed have the condition or disease D when the test result is positive, i.e., $\mathrm{pr}(D|y = 1)$. Likewise, the probability of correctly ruling out the disease when the test is negative is also of interest, i.e., $\mathrm{pr}(\bar{D}|y = 0)$. To calculate these probabilities, called "predictive values" (Galen and Gambino, 1975), the notions of sensitivity and specificity do not suffice. For two diagnostic classes and a binary test, Bayes' theorem states that

$$\begin{aligned} \mathrm{pr}(D|y=1) &= \frac{\mathrm{pr}(D)\ \mathrm{pr}(y = 1|D)}{\mathrm{pr}(D)\ \mathrm{pr}(y = 1|D) + \mathrm{pr}(\bar{D})\ \mathrm{pr}(y = 1|\bar{D})} \\ &= \frac{\mathrm{pr}(D)\ SE(d)}{\mathrm{pr}(D)\ SE(d) + \mathrm{pr}(\bar{D})\ \{1 - SP(d)\}} \end{aligned} \tag{4.2}$$

where $\mathrm{pr}(D)$ denotes the "prior probability" of the illness under consideration in this patient, that is, the physician's degree of belief expressed as a probability, before knowing the result of the laboratory test, that the patient is indeed ill. In some cases, pr(D) might simply be the estimated prevalence of the disease among the population in the area. To simplify notation, let pr(D) $= p$. Since we assumed that the patient belongs either to class D or class $\overline{D}$, pr($\overline{D}$) $= 1 - p$. Then, we rewrite equation (4.2) as

$$\mathrm{pr}(D|y = 1) = \frac{pSE(d)}{pSE(d) + (1 - p)\{1 - SP(d)\}} \tag{4.3}$$

Similarly, we can show that

$$\mathrm{pr}(\overline{D}|y = 0) = \frac{(1 - p)SP(d)}{(1 - p)SP(d) + p\{1 - SE(d)\}} \tag{4.4}$$

Now, let $L(1)$ denote the ratio of the probabilities of a "positive" result ($y = 1$) under each diagnostic class, i.e., $L(1) = \mathrm{pr}(y = 1|D)/\mathrm{pr}(y = 1|\overline{D})$. Then, $L(1) = SE(d)/[1 - SP(d)]$, and we may now write (4.3) in the form

$$\mathrm{pr}(D|y = 1) = \frac{pL(1)}{pL(1) + (1 - p)} \tag{4.5}$$

The ratio $L(1)$ is called the likelihood ratio of the result $y = 1$. Similarly, if we denote by $L(0)$ the likelihood ratio of the negative result $y = 0$, then $L(0) = \mathrm{pr}(y = 0|D)/\mathrm{pr}(y = 0|\overline{D}) = [1 - SE(d)]/SP(d)$, and (4.4) may be written

$$\mathrm{pr}(\overline{D}|y = 0) = \frac{1 - p}{(1 - p) + pL(0)} \tag{4.6}$$

The left-hand side of (4.5) is called the "posterior probability" of illness D in the given patient after a positive test result has been obtained. It is also called the "predictive value" of a positive result ($PV+$). The left-hand side of (4.6) is called the posterior probability of nonillness $\overline{D}$ in the patient after a negative result, or the predictive value of a negative result ($PV-$). Predictive values depend on the particular choice of a cutoff point d, while the prior probability does not.

These predictive values measure the interpretive capabilities of the dichotomized laboratory test, that is, the usefulness of this test to the physician attempting to differentiate between conditions D and $\overline{D}$ in a given patient. When the test is useless in the evaluative sense discussed earlier, $SP(d) = SE(d) = 1/2, L(0) = L(1) = 1, PV+ = p$, while $PV- = 1 - p$. In other words the interpretive probabilities after the test result is known are the same as they were before the test. On the other hand, a very efficient test in terms of specificity and sensitivity may still be poor in its interpretive ability if the prior probability (or prevalence) of the illness is small. Consider, for example, a test with a strong ability to separate populations D and $\overline{D}$ at a given cutoff point d. Suppose $SE(d) = 0.90$ and $SP(d) = 0.95$ for this test, so that $L(1) = 18$ and $L(0) = 0.105$. If the prior probability of the disease is 0.2, then using equation (4.5), $PV+ = (0.2 \times 18)/(0.2 \times 18 + 0.8) = 0.82$, or 82%, while, from equation (4.6), $PV-$ equals 97%. However, if the disease is relatively rare, with prior probability $p = 0.01$, $PV+$ drops to 15% while $PV-$ increases to virtually 100%. In this case, the probability of a false positive result ($1 - PV+$) is quite high, 85%, while a false negative is almost impossible. To reduce the probability of false positive interpretation to less than, say, 30% in this situation, both the sensitivity and specificity of the test would have to exceed 0.995.

Specificity and sensitivity are concepts related to a single laboratory test whose values are dichotomized via a decision point d. This approach has a number of serious drawbacks. First, laboratory tests are often continuous variables with clinical interpretation depending on the actual value of the result. In this case, the dichotomization process may entail a substantial loss of information. Moreover, specificity and sensitivity are then dependent on an arbitrary choice of cutoff point on a basically continuous scale. This may be an advantage in epidemiological studies where one may wish the freedom to weight specificity more heavily than sensitivity, or vice versa. However, the "rubbery" quality of these concepts when X is not a binary variable makes them generally unsuitable for the interpretive use of a specific test value in a given patient. Finally, the extension of specificity and sensitivity to multivariate continuous variables would be quite difficult even for multivariate normal distributions involving complicated multiple integrations.

Our study of the single, dichotomized laboratory test has uncovered one very useful idea, the likelihood ratio. The remainder of this chapter will be devoted to further development of this concept and its application to the interpretation of laboratory tests.

4.4 THE LIKELIHOOD RATIO

As before, the disease state or condition under consideration will be denoted by D, also used to describe the group of patients suffering from the disease. The complementary state, and the group of patients not suffering from D, will be denoted by $\overline{D}$. In general, we will consider a vector of k laboratory or other tests from whose values $(x_1, \ldots, x_k)$, the diagnosis of D is to be made. These tests may be binary, continuous, or even categorical, i.e., discrete with more than two outcomes. Hence the observation vector $\mathbf{X}$ can be a combination of discrete and continuous variables.

In the purely binary case discussed earlier the likelihood ratio was defined as the ratio of two probabilities. For a continuous variable, the ratio would be that of two probability density functions. Since the concept of a probability density function (*pdf*), $f(x)$, is valid for both discrete and continuous variables, we will still use the notation $\text{pr}(\mathbf{x})$, although it is properly restricted to discrete variables only. The likelihood ratio for any observed value of $\mathbf{X}$ (say, $\mathbf{x}_0$) is defined by (Albert, 1982):

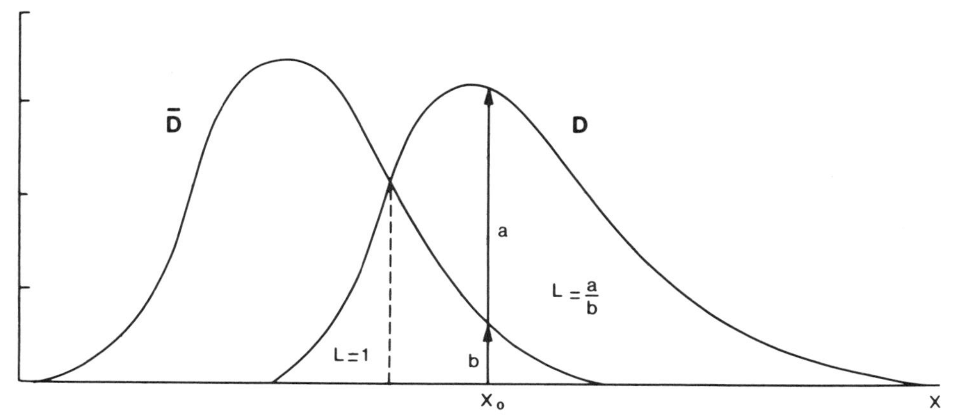

FIGURE 4.3 Likelihood ratio associated with an observed value x_0 of a laboratory test X: $L(x_0) = a/b$, where $a = \text{pr}(x_0|D)$ and $b = \text{pr}(x_0|\overline{D})$.

$$L(\mathbf{x}_0) = \frac{\text{pr}(\mathbf{x}_0|D)}{\text{pr}(\mathbf{x}_0|\overline{D})} \tag{4.7}$$

where $\text{pr}(\mathbf{x}_0|D)$ represents the *pdf* of $\mathbf{X}$ at the point $\mathbf{x}_0$ in the presence of disease D, and $\text{pr}(\mathbf{x}_0|\overline{D})$, the *pdf* of $\mathbf{X}$ at $\mathbf{x}_0$ in the absence of D. Figure 4.3 illustrates the definition of the likelihood ratio when only one continuous laboratory test is considered. The two curves represent the *pdf*'s of X in populations $\overline{D}$ and D, respectively. Following equation (4.7), the likelihood ratio at the point x_0 is a/b. An observed value in the neighborhood of x_0 is more likely to come from group D than $\overline{D}$. In a multivariate situation, $L(\mathbf{x})$ would be defined by the ratio of joint density functions under D and $\overline{D}$.

4.5 PROPERTIES OF THE LIKELIHOOD RATIO

A. For all $\mathbf{x}$, $L(\mathbf{x}) > 0$ since it is the ratio of two positive numbers. Even if $\mathbf{x}_0$ is a multivariate profile, $L(\mathbf{x}_0)$ is always a number, that is, a univariate quantity. It summarizes in a single value the diagnostic implication of the observed profile with respect to the disease considered.

B. A value $L(\mathbf{x}_0) > 1$ signifies that the observed profile is more likely to come from D than $\overline{D}$, and conversely if $L(\mathbf{x}_0) < 1$. As we noted earlier, the value $L = 1$ implies that the observation vector is of no help in distinguishing between the two diagnostic classes. In Figure 4.3, this corresponds to the value where the two distributions intersect (dotted line). A likelihood ratio close to zero rules out the disease D, whereas a very large ratio confirms the presence of D.

C. A likelihood ratio exists for every observed profile; however, different multivariate vectors can lead to the same L-value.

D. When the observation vector $\mathbf{x}^T = (x_1, \ldots, x_k)$ consists of the values of k statistically independent variables, then $L(\mathbf{x})$ becomes the product of the k univariate likelihood ratios. This follows from the fact that the multivariate density function of a set of independent variables is the product of the separate univariate *pdf*'s.

4.6 A GENERAL FORM FOR THE LIKELIHOOD RATIO

Our chief purpose now will be to describe a general equation for the likelihood ratio, applicable to both discrete and continuous variables, either separate or combined in a multivariate profile and distributed in either a multivariate normal or other *pdf*.

The model we adopt for the likelihood ratio is the exponential relation

$$L(\mathbf{x}) = \exp(a_0 + a_1x_1 + \cdots + a_kx_k) \qquad (4.8)$$

where the constant term a_0 and the vector of coefficients $\mathbf{a}^T = (a_1, \ldots, a_k)$ form a set of unknown parameters to be estimated from a sample of data drawn from the nondiseased and diseased populations. Problems related to obtaining a reliable database can be found in Ransohoff and Feinstein (1978). We shall show that this model is appropriate for many laboratory and clinical tests, and, as an example, we apply it to the diagnosis of multiple sclerosis by means of a trivariate test profile.

It is clear, first of all, that equation (4.8) conforms to the properties of likelihood ratios listed above, particularly (*A*) and (*D*). Now let us consider the following special cases.

A. Binary Test

We discussed this case earlier with respect to the dichotomized continuous variable, and noted that $L(0) = [1 - SE(d)]/SP(d)$, and $L(1) = SE(d)/[1 - SP(d)]$. In the dichotomized case, $L(0)$ and $L(1)$, like SE and SP, are functions of the arbitrary cutoff point d. In a genuine binary test, such as the absence or presence of a qualitative characteristic, this arbitrariness would not exist. These equations for $L(0)$ and $L(1)$ may be combined into the exponential model

$$L(x) = \exp(a_0 + a_1 x) \tag{4.9}$$

where

$$\begin{aligned} a_0 &= \log\{(1 - SE)/SP\} \quad \text{and} \\ a_1 &= \log\{SE \cdot SP/(1 - SE)(1 - SP)\} \end{aligned} \tag{4.10}$$

B. Normally Distributed Test

Suppose that the distribution of the laboratory test is normal in both populations $\bar{D}$ and D, with mean values $\mu_{\bar{D}}$ and μ_D, respectively, but common variance σ^2. Using equation (4.7), and writing the likelihood ratio in the exponential form (4.9), we find that

$$\begin{aligned} a_0 &= -{}^1\!/_2(\mu_D^2 - \mu_{\bar{D}}^2)/\sigma^2 \quad \text{and} \\ a_1 &= (\mu_D - \mu_{\bar{D}})/\sigma^2 \end{aligned} \tag{4.11}$$

Estimates of a_0 and a_1 can be obtained by estimating the group means and common variance from the database; substitution in equation (4.9) allows calculation of the likelihood ratio $L(x_0)$ for any observed value x_0.

Suppose now that $\mathbf{X}$ is a vector of k laboratory tests with joint multinormal distribution in both nondiseased and diseased groups. Let $\boldsymbol{\mu}_{\bar{D}}$, $\boldsymbol{\mu}_D$ and $\boldsymbol{\Sigma}$ denote the mean vectors in $\bar{D}$ and D, and the common covariance matrix, respectively. Then, equations (4.9) and (4.11) generalize to

$$L(\mathbf{x}) = \exp(a_0 + \mathbf{a}^T\mathbf{x})$$

where

$$a_0 = -{}^1\!/_2(\boldsymbol{\mu}_D - \boldsymbol{\mu}_{\bar{D}})^T \boldsymbol{\Sigma}^{-1}(\boldsymbol{\mu}_{\bar{D}} + \boldsymbol{\mu}_D) \quad (4.12)$$

and

$$\mathbf{a}^T = (\boldsymbol{\mu}_D - \boldsymbol{\mu}_{\bar{D}})^T\boldsymbol{\Sigma}^{-1} \quad (4.13)$$

Example

In this study (van der Helm and Hische, 1979; and Albert, 1982), three laboratory tests were applied to the differential diagnosis of multiple sclerosis (D) from other neurological diseases ($\bar{D}$). A total of 167 patients were examined, 90 of whom were definitely diagnosed as having multiple sclerosis and 77 classified as suffering from other neurological diseases according to well-defined clinical criteria. The laboratory variables were: (1) cerebrospinal fluid IgG index, defined as the ratio of (IgG in CSF/IgG in serum) to CSF-albumin/S-albumin; (2) presence or absence of monoclonal *Ig* in the cerebrospinal fluid; and (3) the CSF/serum albumin ratio (the denominator of the CSF IgG index). The distributional characteristics of these variables are described in Table 4.2, giving the means and standard deviations of the continuous variables.

TABLE 4.2 Distributional Characteristics of CSF IgG Index, Outcome of Monoclonal Ig in CSF and CSF/S Albumin Ratio in Multiple Sclerosis (D) and in Other Neurological Diseases ($\overline{D}$)

	Multiple sclerosis	
	Absent ($\overline{D}$) ($n = 77$)	Present (D) ($n = 90$)
Laboratory tests:		
X_1: CSF IgG index	0.59 ± 0.23	1.29 ± 0.89
X_2: Presence of monoclonal Ig in CSF		
No (0)	69	20
Yes (1)	8	70
X_3: CSF/S albumin ratio ($\times 10^{-3}$)	7.65 ± 5.41	6.85 ± 3.32

Source: Adapted from Albert (1982).

The second variable, presence ($x_2 = 1$) or absence ($x_2 = 0$) of monoclonal Ig, is the simplest case here. From Table 4.2, $SP = 69/77 = 0.896$, and $SE = 70/90 = 0.778$, from which, using equations (4.10),

$$L(x_2) = \exp(-1.394 + 3.407\, x_2)$$

The likelihood ratios associated with $x_2 = 0$ and $x_2 = 1$ are $L(0) = 0.25$ and $L(1) = 7.50$, respectively. In other words, the presence of monoclonal Ig in the CSF is seven to eight times more frequent in multiple sclerosis than in the other neurological diseases. In contrast, a negative test is found in 1:4 proportion, four times more likely in the nonmultiple sclerosis group.

For the sake of illustration, assume that the distribution of the albumin ratio (x_3) is approximately normal in both patient groups, although with slightly different standard deviations. From Table 4.2, $\bar{x}_{\overline{D}} = 7.65$, $\bar{x}_D = 6.85$, and pooled $s = 4.41$, the square root of the weighted average variance. Using equations (4.11),

$$L(x_3) = \exp(0.298 - 0.041\, x_3)$$

An albumin ratio ($\times\ 10^{-3}$) of 5.0, for example, yields a likelihood ratio $L(x_3) = 1.10$, almost equally likely in both groups. Suppose we had decided not to assume equal variances in each diagnostic class for this variable. Then, under the univariate normal distribution, setting $L(x) = \exp(a_0 + a_1 x + a_2 x^2)$, we find that

$$\begin{aligned} a_0 &= -{}^1\!/_2(\mu_D^2\sigma_{\bar{D}}^2 - \mu_{\bar{D}}^2\sigma_D^2)/(\sigma_D\sigma_{\bar{D}})^2 + \log(\sigma_{\bar{D}}/\sigma_D) \\ a_1 &= (\mu_D\sigma_{\bar{D}}^2 - \mu_{\bar{D}}\sigma_D^2)/(\sigma_D\sigma_{\bar{D}})^2 \\ a_2 &= -{}^1\!/_2(\sigma_{\bar{D}}^2 - \sigma_D^2)/(\sigma_D\sigma_{\bar{D}})^2 \end{aligned} \tag{4.14}$$

Inserting corresponding statistics from Table 4.2, we obtain

$$L(x_3) = \exp(-0.640 + 0.360\, x_3 - 0.0283\, x_3^2)$$

Substituting again for x_3 an observed albumin ratio of 5 yields $L(x_3) = 1.57$, slightly more in favor of the diagnosis of multiple sclerosis but still essentially neutral. The calculation of posterior probabilities, which are the final statistical guides to the diagnostic decision, will be discussed in Section 4.8.

4.7 ESTIMATING THE LIKELIHOOD RATIO FORMULA

Proceeding under the general assumption [equation (4.8)] that $L(\mathbf{x}) = \exp(a_0 + \mathbf{a}^T\mathbf{x})$, the problem of calculating $L(\mathbf{x})$ reduces to estimating the unknown parameters $a_0, a_1, \ldots, a_k$ from available data. In particular, we require a general method that makes no special assumption about the distributional form of the multivariate profile in either diagnostic group.

We shall see in the next chapter that the likelihood ratio method is closely related to another important technique of statistical interpretation, logistic discriminant analysis

(Anderson, 1972). This methodology provides maximum likelihood estimates, say $\hat{a}_0^*$, $\hat{a}_1, \ldots, \hat{a}_k$, for the unknown parameters, but to obtain the estimate $\hat{a}_0$ for $L(\mathbf{x})$ requires an adjustment (Albert, 1982), namely,

$$\hat{a}_0 = \hat{a}_0^* + \log\{n(\overline{D})/n(D)\} \tag{4.15}$$

where $n(D)$ and $n(\overline{D})$ represent the sample sizes from populations D and $\overline{D}$. If $n(\overline{D}) = n(D)$, then $\hat{a}_0^*$ is unaffected. This estimation method is quite general, and unless the exact distribution of $\mathbf{X}$ in the two populations are known, it is recommended.

Example

We applied the logistic estimation method separately to each of the laboratory variables used in the differential diagnosis of multiple sclerosis and obtained the following equations:

1. CSF IgG index: $L(x_1) = \exp(-4.093 + 5.234\, x_1)$
2. Monoclonal Ig in CSF: $L(x_2) = \exp(-1.394 + 3.407\, x_2)$
3. Albumin ratio: $L(x_3) = \exp(0.306 - 0.042\, x_3)$

For the binary test (x_2), the logistic estimation procedure yields exactly the same coefficients as given by equation (4.10). For the albumin ratio, results are in close agreement with the assumption of a normally distributed variable with constant variance [equation (4.11)]. For the CSF IgG index, no relatively simple distributional assumptions can be made, and a general estimation technique like the logistic procedure must be used.

This method also allows estimating the likelihood ratio for any combination of variables, e.g., CSF IgG index (x_1), monoclonal Ig (x_2). For this pair, we estimate

$$L(\mathbf{x}) = \exp(-3.676 + 3.430\, x_1 + 2.333\, x_2) \tag{4.16}$$

For example, an IgG index of 0.79 combined with the absence of monoclonal Ig in the CSF yields $L(\mathbf{x}) = 0.38$; whereas the same IgG index value together with the presence of monoclonal Ig increases the likelihood ratio tenfold to $L(\mathbf{x}) = 3.92$. This result indicates that this pattern is four times more frequent in multiple sclerosis than in the other neurological diseases.

4.8 POSTERIOR PROBABILITY IN THE MULTIVARIATE CASE

The likelihood ratio associated with a vector of laboratory results summarizes into a single index the diagnostic implications of the laboratory and clinical information obtained for the patient. The final statistical calculation to guide decision-making in this situation is the posterior probability (or predictive value) of diagnostic class D in the patient given the vector of results. By extension of Bayes' theorem, we find that

$$\mathrm{pr}(D|\mathbf{x}) = \frac{pL(\mathbf{x})}{(1 - p) + pL(\mathbf{x})} \quad \text{and} \qquad \mathrm{pr}(\overline{D}|\mathbf{x}) = \frac{1 - p}{(1 - p) + pL(\mathbf{x})} \tag{4.17}$$

where p, as before, is the prior probability, or degree of belief, for diagnostic class D. Thus, equations (4.17) extend the concept of predictive values from binary and dichotomized tests to any laboratory profile $\mathbf{x}^T = (x_1, \ldots, x_k)$. Observe that from (4.17) the prior odds ratio $r = p/(1 - p)$ and the posterior odds ratio $R(\mathbf{x}) = \mathrm{pr}(D|\mathbf{x})/\mathrm{pr}(\overline{D}|\mathbf{x})$ are related by the equation

$$R(\mathbf{x}) = rL(\mathbf{x}) \tag{4.18}$$

The value given to the prior probability in equations (4.17) depends on the clinical context. In screening randomly for a disease, p would be the prevalence of the disease in the population screened. This might be quite low. Higher values of p obtain where the diagnosis is suspected, but there is uncertainty, and laboratory tests are ordered to reduce this uncertainty. The stronger the initial suspicion, the higher the clinician should set the value of p, which then, of course, will vary with the individual patient.

Equations (4.17) show that only the prior probability and the likelihood ratio are needed to calculate the posterior probability. This posterior probability may in turn become a new prior if additional test results or other information becomes available, provided that a likelihood ratio for this new information can be determined. As mentioned earlier, different values of $\mathbf{x}$ may lead to the same likelihood ratio and, therefore, the same posterior probability.

Example

Consider the diagnosis of multiple sclerosis in a patient presenting an IgG index of 0.79 and showing monoclonal immunoglobulins in the CSF. We calculated above that in this case, the likelihood ratio is 3.92. Assuming a prior probability of 0.60, equation (4.17) gives a posterior probability of 0.85, almost confirming the diagnosis.

4.9 THE LIKELIHOOD RATIO AS A GENERAL INDEX OF DIAGNOSTIC EFFICIENCY

We have been discussing the likelihood ratio as a means of interpreting a vector of observations from a patient to help resolve a problem in differential diagnosis. It can also be used to judge the general diagnostic efficiency of a proposed set of laboratory or clinical variables; in other words, as an index of specificity and sensitivity applicable to a multivariate profile. This becomes possible because, through the likelihood ratio, a multidimensional space is reduced to the domain of a single variable.

As with any measure of specificity or sensitivity, this use of $L(\mathbf{x})$ will depend on an arbitrary choice of cutoff point. In the case of $L(\mathbf{x})$, however, in contrast to a single laboratory test, a suitable choice can be made independently of any distribution of observed values within a diagnostic class. The point $L(\mathbf{x}) = 1$ represents the most attractive divider because a vector of observations for which $L(\mathbf{x}) = 1$ does not favor either diagnostic class. More explicitly, when $L(\mathbf{x}) = 1$, the posterior probability remains exactly equal to the prior probability. Therefore, if we define a "generalized" specificity and sensitivity by the expressions

$$\begin{aligned} SP &= \mathrm{pr}\{L(\mathbf{x}) \leq 1 | \overline{D}\} \\ SE &= \mathrm{pr}\{L(\mathbf{x}) > 1 | D\} \end{aligned} \tag{4.19}$$

we will have a general quantitative measure of the differential diagnostic efficiency of profile $\mathbf{X}$ with respect to disease D.

For example, to appraise the joint ability of CSF IgG index (x_1) and the demonstration of monoclonal Ig in the CSF (x_2) to diagnose multiple sclerosis, we calculated the likelihood ratio based on these two tests [equation (4.16)] for each of the 167 patients in the foregoing study and classified these ratios in a 2 × 2 table (Table 4.3) using the cutoff point $L = 1$.

TABLE 4.3 Cross-classification of 167 Patients According to True Diagnosis (Absence or Presence of Multiple Sclerosis) and Likelihood Ratio Calculated from CSF IgG Index and Demonstration of Monoclonal Ig in the CSF [Equation (4.16)]: Generalized Specificity and Sensitivity

		Multiple sclerosis	
		Absent ($n = 77$)	Present ($n = 90$)
Likelihood	$L \leqslant 1$	67	14
ratio $L(\mathbf{x})$	$L > 1$	10	76

Source: Adapted from Albert (1982).

Estimated specificity was 67/77 = 0.87 and sensitivity 76/90 = 0.84. This represents an improvement in sensitivity over x_2 alone, for which $SE = 0.78$, but a decline in specificity since $SP = 0.90$ for x_2 alone. Assuming a prevalence of about 50% multiple sclerotic patients among the group studied, the addition of CSF IgG index does not improve, in fact slightly weakens, the predictive value of the presence of monoclonal Ig.

4.10
A LITTLE MORE ABOUT LIKELIHOOD RATIOS

A. Confidence Intervals

When the maximum likelihood estimates of the coefficients in the likelihood ratio equation (4.8) are calculated, the asymptotic dispersion matrix **V** (the matrix of variances and covariances) of these estimates is also estimated ($\hat{\mathbf{V}}$). An adjustment to the variance of the estimate of a_0 may be needed. If $\hat{a}_0^*$ denotes the maximum likelihood estimate, and $\hat{a_0}$ the adjusted estimate [see equation (4.15)], then (Anderson, 1972)

$$\text{var}(\hat{a}_0) = \text{var}(\hat{a}_0^*) - 1/n(\overline{D}) - 1/n(D) \tag{4.20}$$

The matrix $\hat{\mathbf{V}}$ enables one to determine confidence limits not only for the unknown parameters $a_0, a_1, \ldots, a_k$, but also for the likelihood ratio itself. A β-confidence interval for $L(\mathbf{x})$ is given by the limits

$$\exp\{\log \hat{L}(\mathbf{x}) \pm z(1 - \beta/2)\text{v}(\mathbf{x})\} \tag{4.21}$$

where $\hat{\text{L}}(\mathbf{x})$ is the calculated likelihood ratio, $z(1 - \beta/2)$ is the upper β/2 percentage point of the standard normal distribution, and $v^2(\mathbf{x}) = (1,\mathbf{x}^T)\hat{\mathbf{V}}(1,\mathbf{x}^T)^T$ the estimated asymptotic variance of $\hat{a}_0 + \hat{a}_1x_1 + \cdots + \hat{a}_kx_k$. For example, if there are only two variables $\mathbf{x}^T = (x_1,x_2)$, then

$$v^2(\mathbf{x}) = V_{11}x_1^2 + V_{22}x_2^2 + 2V_{12}x_1x_2 + 2V_{01}x_1 + 2V_{02}x_2 + V_{00}, \text{ where } V_{ij} = \text{cov}(\hat{a}_i,\hat{a}_j), (i,j = 0,1,2).$$

[See also Gruemer et al. (1984) for more detail.]

Example

Referring to the diagnosis of multiple sclerosis and the examples discussed in this chapter, we found

$$\hat{\mathbf{V}} = \begin{bmatrix} 0.4062 & & \\ -0.5242 & 0.7801 & \\ -0.0007 & -0.1152 & 0.2522 \end{bmatrix}$$

Thus, applying the formula above, we have

1. CSF IgG index $= 0.79$ and absence of monoclonal Ig in *CSF* $(x_2 = 0)$
   $L(\mathbf{x}) = 0.38$ (0.95 confidence interval:0.23 – 0.63)
2. CSF IgG index $= 0.79$ and presence of monoclonal Ig in CSF $(x_2 = 1)$
   $L(\mathbf{x}) = 3.92$ (0.95 confidence interval: 1.92 – 8.03)

The first case suggests that at the 5% critical level, $L < 1$, whereas for the second profile observed, $L > 1$.

B. Determination of the Point of Equal Likelihood

In the case of a single quantitative test, it is of interest to determine the value $x = d$ for which the likelihood ratio is equal to unity. Since $L(d) = 1$, $\text{pr}(d|\overline{D}) = \text{pr}(d|D)$, so that $x = d$ marks the point on the scale of test values where the two *pdf* s intersect (Figure 4.3). Using the exponential model for $L(x)$,

$$L(d) = \exp(a_0 + a_1 d) = 1 \qquad \text{so that}$$
$$a_0 + a_1 d = 0 \qquad \text{or} \tag{4.22}$$
$$d = -a_0/a_1$$

In practice, d would be estimated by $-\hat{a}_0/\hat{a}_1$.

Example

The likelihood ratio formula for the CSF IgG index was found to be $L(x_1) = \exp(-4.093 + 5.234\ x_1)$, so that $d = 4.093/5.234 = 0.78$. This value is equally likely in both groups $\overline{D}$ and D. Any IgG index above 0.78, yielding a likelihood ratio $L > 1$, is more likely in the multiple sclerosis patients, while any index below 0.78 is more frequent in patients with other neurological disorders. It may be noted that the upper reference limit for the IgG index in healthy subjects is 0.62 (van der Helm and Hische, 1979).

C. Diagnostic Effectiveness and Test Selection

Clearly, the likelihood ratio formula (4.8) can be derived for any individual test or combination of tests. However, this will be useless if the diseased and nondiseased populations overlap substantially, since in this case $L = 1$ for almost every result. Likewise, if some variables of a profile contain repetitious information, it may be preferable to discard these variables and to determine a simpler equation for the likelihood ratio.

The best way to proceed would be (1) to assess and test the individual diagnostic ability of each constituent of the profile $\mathbf{X}$ with respect to the disease D; and (2) to select the best subset of variables for discriminating between diseased and nondiseased populations. Under the general model (4.8), the logistic discrimination method described in Chapter 5 provides a satisfactory solution to this problem. In both cases, the statistics used are distributed as a χ^2-test on one degree of freedom. The larger the χ^2-value, the better the univariate diagnostic ability or the contribution of the variable added to those already selected (see Section 5.5).

Example

The individual diagnostic ability of the three laboratory tests given in Table 4.2 for multiple sclerosis was obtained by applying logistic discrimination to the patients' data. The demonstration of monoclonal Ig in the CSF ($\chi^2 = 84.1$, 1 df, $p < 0.001$) was found to be highly significant and slightly superior to CSF IgG index ($\chi^2 = 82.7$, 1 df, $p < 0.001$). The chi-square value ($\chi^2 = 1.4$) for the CSF/S albumin ratio was not statistically significant, indicating that the likelihood ratio equation for this test is irrelevant. When combining variables X_1 and X_2 to obtain equation (4.16), we conclude that the addition of IgG index to the electrophoretic test significantly improved the discrimination between multiple sclerosis and other neurological diseases ($\chi^2 = 22.4$, 1 df, $p < 0.001$).

REFERENCES

Albert, A. (1981). Atypicality indices as reference values for laboratory data. *Am J. Clin. Path. 76,* 421–425.

Albert, A. (1982). On the use and computation of likelihood ratios in clinical chemistry. *Clin. Chem. 5,* 1113–1119.

Anderson, J. A. (1972). Separate sample logistic discrimination. *Biometrika 59*, 19–35.

Galen, R. S., and Gambino, S. R. (1975). *Beyond Normality: The Predictive Value and Efficiency of Medical Diagnoses.* Wiley, New York.

Gruemer, H. S., Miller, W. G., Chinchilli, V. M., Leshner, R. T., Hassler, C. R., Blasco, P. A., Nance, W. E., and Goldsmith, B. M. (1984). Are reference limits for serum creatine kinase valid in the detection of the carrier state for Duchenne muscular dystrophy? *Clin. Chem. 30*, 724–730.

Hanley, J. A., and McNeil, B. J. (1983). A method of comparing the areas under receiver operating characteristic curves derived from the same cases. *Radiology 148*, 839–843.

McNeil, B. J., and Hanley, J. A. (1984). Statistical approaches to the analysis of receiver operating characteristic (*ROC*) curves. *Med. Decis. Making 4*, 137–150.

Ransohoff, D. F., and Feinstein, A. R. (1978). Problem of spectrum and bias in evaluating the efficacy of diagnostic tests. *N. Engl. J. Med. 299*, 926–930.

Swets, J. A. (1979). *ROC* analysis applied to the evaluation of medical imaging techniques. *Invest. Radiol. 14*, 109–121.

van der Helm, H. J., and Hische, E. A. (1979). Application of Bayes' theorem to results of quantitative clinical determinations. *Clin. Chem. 25*, 985–988.

Yerushalmy, J. (1947). Statistical problems in assessing methods of medical diagnosis with special reference to X-ray techniques. *Public Health Rep. 62*, 1432–1449.

5

Differential Diagnosis: Several Categories

5.1
INTRODUCTION

The use of a laboratory profile to distinguish between nondiseased and diseased populations by means of the likelihood ratio can be generalized to a differential diagnosis among several diseases. The statistical methods enabling a patient to be classified into one of a set of diseases (or diseased groups) on the basis of a laboratory profile all depend on a general methodology called discriminant analysis. The comprehensive description of discriminant analysis falls beyond the scope of this book, and the reader can always refer to specialized textbooks if needed (e.g., Anderson, 1958; Cacoullos, 1973; and Lachenbruch, 1975). In this chapter, we will describe two discriminant techniques for interpretation of multivariate laboratory data with particular emphasis on likelihood ratios. Either of these methods should resolve most differential diagnostic problems encountered in practice. The first is based on multinormal assumptions and is called classical linear discriminant analysis. The second method, logistic discrimination, is applicable to mixed variable sets (binary or continuous-valued tests) and is therefore more relaxed about distributional assumptions. Unavoidably, the material in this chapter uses the notation of vectors and matrices. As far as possible, however, we illustrate the methods by examples for the two- or three-group case. See also Solberg (1978) for a comprehensive review of the subject in clinical chemistry.

5.2
PROBLEM FORMULATION

We denote by $D_1, \ldots, D_g$ the g diseased categories under consideration, and by $p_1, \ldots, p_g$ the corresponding prior probabilities. Since every patient is supposed to belong to one of these categories, $p_1 + \cdots + p_g = 1$. Let $\mathbf{X}^T = (X_1, \ldots, X_k)$ be a k-dimensional laboratory test battery, no restriction being made at present about the nature of these tests.

The statistical problem to be resolved is the following: On the basis of a laboratory profile $\mathbf{x}_0$, to what disease group should the patient be allocated? Further, how does the observed profile $\mathbf{x}_0$ revise the prior probabilities $p_1, \ldots, p_g$? As mentioned earlier, any attempt at such interpretation of data is likely to fail if the distributions of laboratory profiles under the various diseases overlap substantially. This relates to the problem of laboratory profile evaluation, discussed later in this chapter. Again, we note the distinction between the *evaluation* of a test profile $\mathbf{X}$ (i.e., its ability to discriminate among a set of specific diseases) and the *interpretation* (i.e., classification) of an observed profile $\mathbf{x}_0$ for a particular patient. Modern theory of discriminant analysis provides a complete solution to both discrimination and classification problems.

The general principle is as follows: Let E be the space of all possible values of the laboratory profile $\mathbf{X}$; for a single continuous-valued variable, E is generally the set of positive values. By definition, an allocation rule, noted δ, can be considered as a partition of the space E into g regions $R_1, \ldots, R_g$ such that if $\mathbf{x}_0$ falls into the region R_i ($\mathbf{x}_0 \in R_i$), then the patient is allocated to disease D_i. Recall that, by definition of a partition, the regions $R_1, \ldots, R_g$ are disjoint (i.e., they share no points in common) and their union $R_1 + \cdots + R_g = E$ (see Figure 5.1). Thus any observed profile $\mathbf{x}_0$ must necessarily fall into one and only one region, and thus be allocated to one and only one group.

There are many ways to partition the E space into g regions (often an infinity); consequently there are many different allocation rules δ. Any allocation rule necessarily entails misclassification; thus, some patients suffering from disease D_i can yield laboratory profiles that fall in the region R_j ($j \neq i$) and therefore be diagnosed as suffering from illness D_j. In other words, the population distributions overlap to some extent. Figure 5.2 illustrates the example of two different classification rules. An optimal classification rule δ^* is one for which the misclassification rate is minimal. This is the kind

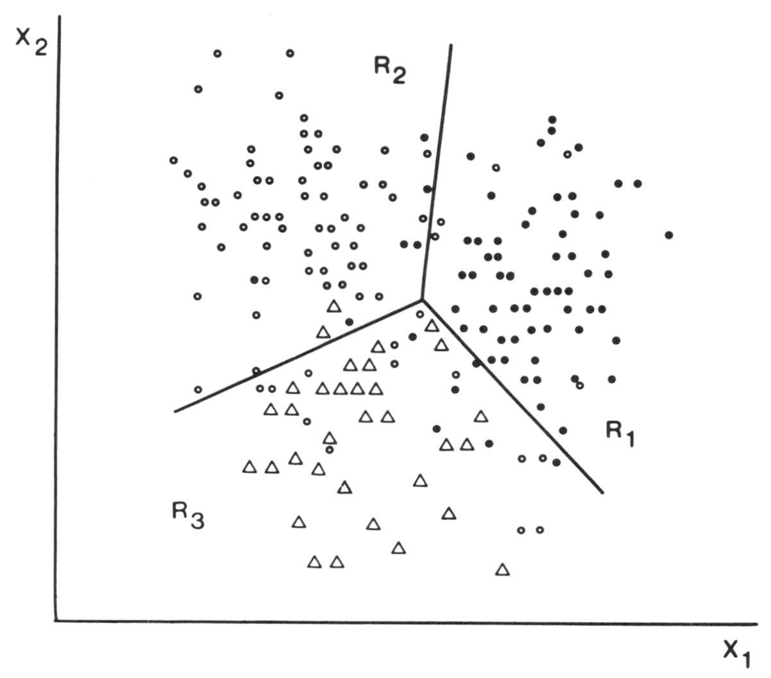

FIGURE 5.1 Partition of a two-dimensional observation-space $E = \{x: x_1 \geq 0, x_2 \geq 0\}$ into three allocation regions R_1, R_2, and R_3.

of allocation rule one is seeking, and the associated error rate provides an estimation of the degree of overlapping of the various disease groups under consideration.

Classification rules are rather rigid since they always allocate an observation $\mathbf{x}_0$ to only one group, that corresponding to the region R to which $\mathbf{x}_0$ belongs. For example, when looking at Figure 5.1, we may imagine an observation $\mathbf{x}_0$ falling close to the borderline between R_1 and R_2, yet on the R_1 side. Although this patient is diagnosed as having disease D_1, disease D_2 cannot be definitely ruled out. Therefore, we propose

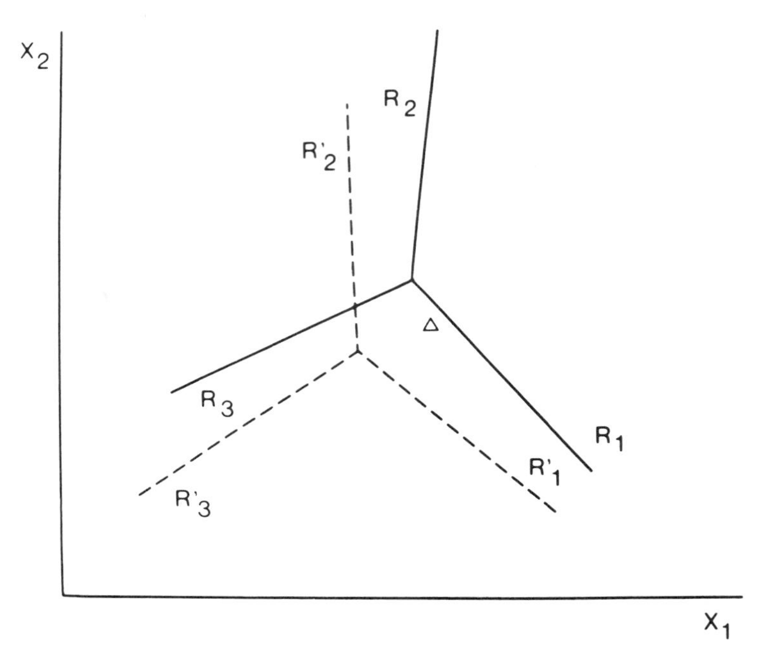

Figure 5.2 Two different partitionings of the observation-space $E = \{\mathbf{x}: x_1 \geq 0, x_2 \geq 0\}$ into three allocation regions. For the decision rule δ (solid lines), the observed vector $\mathbf{x}_0$ (triangle) is classified into group D_3, while for decision rule δ' (dotted lines), $\mathbf{x}_0$ should be allocated to group D_1.

to complete this information by calculating the posterior probabilities of belonging to each of the diseased categories. The final decision, of course, is left to the attending physician. We determine for each observed profile $\mathbf{x}_0$ a vector of posterior probabilities, $\mathbf{P}^T = (P_1, \ldots, P_g)$, where $P_i = \text{pr}(D_i|\mathbf{x}_0)$ $(i = 1, \ldots, g)$ and $P_1 + \cdots + P_g = 1$. In the two-group case, since $P_1 + P_2 = 1$, only one needs to be determined. The discrimination methods described below allow us to resolve the differential diagnostic problem through allocation rules and posterior probabilities.

5.3 POSTERIOR PROBABILITIES AND LIKELIHOOD RATIOS

Given the prior probabilities $p_1, \ldots, p_g$ of the g diseased categories and the probability distributions of the laboratory profile $\mathbf{X}$ in each disease, namely $\mathrm{pr}(\mathbf{x}|D_1), \ldots, \mathrm{pr}(\mathbf{x}|D_g)$, we can calculate the posterior probabilities (or predictive values) using Bayes' theorem:

$$\mathrm{pr}(D_i|\mathbf{x}) = \frac{p_i \mathrm{pr}(\mathbf{x}|D_i)}{p_1 \mathrm{pr}(\mathbf{x}|D_1) + \cdots + p_g \mathrm{pr}(\mathbf{x}|D_g)} \qquad (i = 1, \ldots, g) \tag{5.1}$$

for which all elements have been defined. Dividing both terms of the ratio on the right-hand side of equation (5.1) by $\mathrm{pr}(\mathbf{x}|D_g)$ we obtain an alternative expression for the posterior probabilities, namely

$$\mathrm{pr}(D_i|\mathbf{x}) = \frac{p_i L_{ig}(\mathbf{x})}{p_1 L_{1g}(\mathbf{x}) + \cdots + p_g L_{gg}(\mathbf{x})} \tag{5.2}$$

in which

$$L_{ig}(\mathbf{x}) = \frac{\mathrm{pr}(\mathbf{x}|D_i)}{\mathrm{pr}(\mathbf{x}|D_g)} \tag{5.3}$$

represents the likelihood ratio of the multivariate observation $\mathbf{x}$ for diseased populations D_i and D_g, a concept defined in Chapter 4. In deriving (5.2), we implicitly assume that D_g is the base or reference group to which all other populations are compared. This is just a convention; any group could be used. Equation (5.2) relates posterior probabilities to prior probabilities and likelihood ratios. Observe that only $g - 1$ likelihood ratios need to be known, since $L_{gg}(\mathbf{x}) = 1$.

Examples

For the two-group problem (D_1 and D_2), only one likelihood ratio $L_{12}(\mathbf{x})$ has to be available. When three diseases are under consideration, D_1, D_2, and D_3, two likelihood ratios suffice, $L_{13}(\mathbf{x})$ and $L_{23}(\mathbf{x})$, and equation (5.2) becomes

$$\text{pr}(D_1|\mathbf{x}) = \frac{p_1 L_{13}(\mathbf{x})}{p_1 L_{13}(\mathbf{x}) + p_2 L_{23}(\mathbf{x}) + p_3}$$

$$\text{pr}(D_2|\mathbf{x}) = \frac{p_2 L_{23}(\mathbf{x})}{p_1 L_{13}(\mathbf{x}) + p_2 L_{23}(\mathbf{x}) + p_3}$$

$$\text{pr}(D_3|\mathbf{x}) = \frac{p_3}{p_1 L_{13}(\mathbf{x}) + p_2 L_{23}(\mathbf{x}) + p_3}$$

From knowledge of the $g - 1$ likelihood ratios (5.3), any other likelihood ratio can be derived. Thus, the likelihood ratio of $\mathbf{x}$ for groups D_n and D_m is obtained as follows:

$$L_{nm}(\mathbf{x}) = \frac{\text{pr}(D_n|\mathbf{x})}{\text{pr}(D_m|\mathbf{x})} = \left(\frac{\text{pr}(D_n|\mathbf{x})}{\text{pr}(D_g|\mathbf{x})}\right)\left(\frac{\text{pr}(D_g|\mathbf{x})}{\text{pr}(D_m|\mathbf{x})}\right)$$

from which

$$L_{nm}(\mathbf{x}) = \frac{L_{ng}(\mathbf{x})}{L_{mg}(\mathbf{x})} \tag{5.4}$$

For example, when $g = 3$,

$$L_{12}(\mathbf{x}) = \frac{L_{13}(\mathbf{x})}{L_{23}(\mathbf{x})}$$

It can be proven that the optimal partition of the observation space E, or equivalently the optimal diagnostic rule δ^* (in the sense of minimizing the overall error rate), is obtained by allocating an observation $\mathbf{x}$ to the diseased group for which the posterior probability is the largest. Formally, the multivariate observation $\mathbf{x}$ is allocated to group D_i if and only if

$$\mathrm{pr}(D_i|\mathbf{x}) \geq \mathrm{pr}(D_j|\mathbf{x}) \qquad (j = 1, \ldots, g) \tag{5.5}$$

In practice, all we need is a method allowing for the calculation of posterior probabilities, or even of likelihood ratios, for once we have such a device, we can use the optimal classification (5.5).

There are at least two possible approaches to this goal. The traditional one consists of assuming that the group-conditional distributions $\mathrm{pr}(\mathbf{x}|D_i)$, $(i = 1, \ldots, g)$ are multinormal. Another way to proceed is to make a parametric assumption about the posterior probabilities (e.g., logistic model). Many nonparametric methods (Fukunaga, 1972) also exist but will not be discussed here.

5.4 NORMAL LINEAR DISCRIMINANT ANALYSIS

A. The Multinormal Model

Let us assume that the probability distribution of the laboratory profile $\mathbf{X}$ in all disease categories is multivariate normal, with different means $\boldsymbol{\mu}_1, \ldots, \boldsymbol{\mu}_g$ but common covariance matrix $\boldsymbol{\Sigma}$. That is,

$$\mathrm{pr}(\mathbf{x}|D_i) = (2\pi)^{-1/2k}|\boldsymbol{\Sigma}|^{1/2}\exp\{-1/2(\mathbf{x} - \boldsymbol{\mu}_i)^T\boldsymbol{\Sigma}^{-1}(\mathbf{x} - \boldsymbol{\mu}_i)\} \tag{5.6}$$
$$(i = 1, \ldots, g)$$

Then the likelihood ratios (5.3) become, after substitution of (5.6),

$$L_{ig}(\mathbf{x}) = \frac{(2\pi)^{k/2}|\boldsymbol{\Sigma}|^{-1/2}\exp\{-{}^1/_2(\mathbf{x} - \boldsymbol{\mu}_i)^T\boldsymbol{\Sigma}^{-1}(\mathbf{x} - \boldsymbol{\mu}_i)\}}{(2\pi)^{k/2}|\boldsymbol{\Sigma}|^{-1/2}\exp\{-{}^1/_2(\mathbf{x} - \boldsymbol{\mu}_g)^T\boldsymbol{\Sigma}^{-1}(\mathbf{x} - \boldsymbol{\mu}_g)\}}$$
$$= \exp\{{}^1/_2(\mathbf{x} - \boldsymbol{\mu}_g)^T\boldsymbol{\Sigma}^{-1}(\mathbf{x} - \boldsymbol{\mu}_g){}^1/_2(\mathbf{x} - \boldsymbol{\mu}_i)^T\boldsymbol{\Sigma}^{-1}(\mathbf{x} - \boldsymbol{\mu}_i)\}$$

After several simplifications, we obtain

$$L_{ig}(\mathbf{x}) = \exp(a_{0i} + \mathbf{a}_i^T\mathbf{x}) \tag{5.7}$$

where

$$a_{0i} = -{}^1/_2(\boldsymbol{\mu}_i - \boldsymbol{\mu}_g)^T\boldsymbol{\Sigma}^{-1}(\boldsymbol{\mu}_i + \boldsymbol{\mu}_g)$$

and

$$\mathbf{a}_i^T = (\boldsymbol{\mu}_i - \boldsymbol{\mu}_g)^T\boldsymbol{\Sigma}^{-1} \tag{5.8}$$

We retrieve the exponential form of the likelihood ratio developed in Chapter 4. Notice that a_{0i} is a scalar, whereas $\mathbf{a}_i^T = (a_{1i}, \ldots, a_{ki})$ is a k-dimensional vector. It is obvious that when $i = g$, $a_{0g} = 0$ and $\mathbf{a}_g = \mathbf{0}$.

Substituting equations (5.7) in the posterior probabilities (5.2), we obtain

$$\mathrm{pr}(D_i|\mathbf{x}) = \frac{\exp\{a_{0i} + \log(p_i/p_g) + \mathbf{a}_i^T\mathbf{x}\}}{\sum_{j=1}^{g}\exp\{a_{0j} + \log(p_j/p_g) + \mathbf{a}_j^T\mathbf{x}\}} \quad (i = 1, \ldots, g) \tag{5.9}$$

The relations (5.9) are remarkable, expressing the posterior probabilities as functions of simple linear combinations of the variables. They lead to what is called "normal linear discriminant analysis." The expressions

$$1_i(\mathbf{x}) = a_{0i} + \log(p_i/p_g) + \mathbf{a}_i^T\mathbf{x} \tag{5.10}$$

are usually called the linear discriminant functions.

The classification rule (5.5) where the posterior probabilities are replaced by their analytic expression (5.9) now becomes

$$\text{Allocate observation } \mathbf{x} \text{ to group } D_i \text{ if } 1_i(\mathbf{x}) \geq 1_j(\mathbf{x}) \quad (j = 1, \ldots, g) \tag{5.11}$$

Examples

To illustrate the results above, consider again the classical situation of differentiating between two diseases D_1 and D_2. Since there is only one likelihood ratio $L_{12}(\mathbf{x})$, or simply $L(\mathbf{x})$, equation (5.8) yields (dropping the subscript i)

$$L(\mathbf{x}) = \exp(a_0 + \mathbf{a}^T\mathbf{x})$$

where

$$a_0 = -{}^1\!/_2(\boldsymbol{\mu}_1 - \boldsymbol{\mu}_2)^T\boldsymbol{\Sigma}^{-1}(\boldsymbol{\mu}_1 + \boldsymbol{\mu}_2)$$
$$\mathbf{a}^T = (\boldsymbol{\mu}_1 - \boldsymbol{\mu}_2)^T\,\boldsymbol{\Sigma}^{-1}$$

a result which we found previously. Applying the classification rule (5.11) above, we obtain:

$$\begin{aligned}\text{Allocate } \mathbf{x} \text{ to disease } & D_1 \text{ if } 1(\mathbf{x}) \leq 0 \\ \text{to disease } & D_2 \text{ if } 1(\mathbf{x}) > 0\end{aligned}$$

where the linear discriminant function

$$1(\mathbf{x}) = a_0 + \log\left[\frac{(1 - p)}{p}\right] + a_1x_1 + \cdots + a_kx_k \tag{5.12}$$

and $p = \text{pr}(D_2)$.

Consider now the interpretation of a laboratory profile with respect to three diseases D_1, D_2, and D_3. Then there are two discriminant functions:

$$l_1(\mathbf{x}) = a_{01} + \log(p_1/p_3) + a_1^T\mathbf{x}$$
$$l_2(\mathbf{x}) = a_{02} + \log(p_2/p_3) + a_2^T\mathbf{x}$$

and the allocation rule (5.11) consists of allocating a patient to

disease D_1, if $l_1(\mathbf{x}) \geq l_2(\mathbf{x})$ and $l_1(\mathbf{x}) \geq 0$

disease D_2, if $l_2(\mathbf{x}) \geq l_1(\mathbf{x})$ and $l_2(\mathbf{x}) \geq 0$

disease D_3, if $0 \geq l_1(\mathbf{x})$ and $0 \geq l_2(\mathbf{x})$

Provided the a-coefficients and the prior probabilities are known, $l_1(\mathbf{x})$ and $l_2(\mathbf{x})$ can be calculated for any $\mathbf{x}$ and the interpretation of the profile is simple using the rule above.

B. Estimation of the Linear Discriminant Functions

In order to be able to use the discriminant method and calculate the posterior probabilities for laboratory data interpretation, we have to estimate the unknown parameters a_{0i} and $\mathbf{a}_i$ $(i = 1, \ldots, g)$ in equation (5.9). There are $(g - 1) + k(g - 1) = (g - 1)(k + 1)$ such parameters, since a_{0g} and the vector $\mathbf{a}_g$ are zero, by definition.

Now the a-coefficients are functions of the population parameters, $\boldsymbol{\mu}_1, \ldots, \boldsymbol{\mu}_g$ and $\boldsymbol{\Sigma}$ [see equation (5.8)]. Estimation of the mean vectors $\boldsymbol{\mu}_i$ and the covariance matrix $\boldsymbol{\Sigma}$ is straightforward, provided a random sample of patients is available from each diseased group D_i. Let n_i denote the size of the sample of patients with disease D_i and $\mathbf{x}_{ij}$, the observation vector of the jth patient with disease D_i. Then

$$\bar{\mathbf{x}}_i = \sum_{j=1}^{n_i} \mathbf{x}_{ij}/n_i$$

$$\mathbf{S} = \frac{(n_1 - 1)\mathbf{S}_1 + \cdots + (n_g - 1)\mathbf{S}_g}{n_1 + \cdots + n_g - g} = \frac{\sum_{i=1}^{g} (n_i - 1)\,\mathbf{S}_i}{n - g}$$

where

$$n = n_1 + n_2 + \cdots + n_g$$

$$\mathbf{S}_i = \frac{\sum_{j=1}^{n_i} (\mathbf{x}_{ij} - \bar{\mathbf{x}}_i)(\mathbf{x}_{ij} - \bar{\mathbf{x}}_i)^T}{n_i - 1}$$

Thus,

$$\begin{aligned} \hat{a}_{0i} &= -\tfrac{1}{2}(\bar{\mathbf{x}}_i - \bar{\mathbf{x}}_g)^T \mathbf{S}^{-1}(\bar{\mathbf{x}}_i + \bar{\mathbf{x}}_g) \\ \hat{\mathbf{a}}_i^T &= (\bar{\mathbf{x}}_i - \bar{\mathbf{x}}_g)^T \mathbf{S}^{-1} \qquad (i = 1, \ldots, g) \end{aligned} \tag{5.13}$$

In general, the prior probabilities p_i are either known or estimated from another source. However, if the sample of n patients is drawn randomly from the mixture of the diseases $D_1 + \cdots + D_g$, then the p_i's can be estimated by the sample proportions $\hat{p}_i = n_i/n$, $(i = 1, \ldots, g)$.

C. Variable Selection

When we allocate patients into one of g possible diseased categories $D_1, \ldots, D_g$ on the basis of a k-test laboratory profile $\mathbf{X}^T = (X_1, \ldots, X_k)$, the question often arises of how to select from among the tests those that are really needed for the diagnostic problem. Indeed, some of the tests may be useless for the problem considered, i.e., they do not discriminate among the g diseases. Other tests are good discriminators, but when combined, they contribute repetitious information because they are highly correlated. All but a selected one or two of such variables could be omitted because they bring no significant additional diagnostic information. This would simplify the original profile and at the same time might lower laboratory costs.

To answer the problem of variable selection, we need a statistical method that enables us to discard useless and redundant tests, retaining only those with the best joint diagnostic ability. In other words, we ought to find among the k tests $X_1, \ldots, X_k$ the best subset of tests in terms of diagnostic efficiency. Clearly, the number of possible subsets to investigate becomes intractably large as k increases. For instance, for a 10-test profile, there are 1023 such subsets! In general, the number of possible combinations is $2^k - 1$. For $k = 20$, there are 1,048,575 combinations! To overcome this difficulty, we describe a method that long experience has shown to provide a satisfactory solution to the problem of variable selection. It is called the stepwise variable selection technique. This technique selects the variables one at a time, starting with the best one, until no significant improvement occurs in diagnostic ability. The principle of the method may be outlined as follows:

(i) Univariate diagnostic ability. For each variable X_i ($i = 1, \ldots, k$) of the profile $\mathbf{X}$, we apply the discriminant analysis method described in this section and measure its diagnostic ability by an F-test* on $g - 1$ and $n - g$ degrees of freedom. This enables one to rank the k variables in decreasing order of diagnostic ability. The corresponding values of the F-test tell which variables are statistically significant discriminators, e.g., at the 5% significance level. Denote by Z_1 the variable with the highest diagnostic ability.

(ii) Selection of the best variable combination. Consider first all pairs of variables (Z_1,X_i) consisting of the variable Z_1 defined above and any of the $k - 1$ remaining variables. The increase in diagnostic ability can be measured each time by an F-test on $g - 1$ and $n - g - 1$ degrees of freedom. Denote by Z_2 the variable leading to the largest increase, i.e., to the highest F-value.

Repeat the same procedure for all triplets (Z_1,Z_2,X_i), where X_i is any of the $k - 2$ remaining variables, for all quadruplets,

---

*The F-criterion results from one-way analysis of variance to test the null hypothesis of equality of mean values in the g-groups considered.

and so forth. In general at step s, the F-test has $g - 1$ and $n - g - s + 1$ degrees of freedom. The stepwise process stops when a subset $(Z_1, \ldots, Z_{k'})$ is found such that adding any of the $k - k'$ remaining variables produces no significant improvement in the diagnostic ability, i.e., none of the F-values exceed the corresponding 5% critical level.

D. Medical Application: Differential Diagnosis of Liver Disease by Means of an Enzyme Profile

To illustrate the methodology, we applied multinormal discrimination to enzyme data collected from 218 patients with liver diseases (Plomteux, 1980). The complete data set is listed in Appendix I. Four diseases are considered: acute viral hepatitis (D_1: 57 patients); persistent chronic hepatitis (D_2: 44 patients); aggressive chronic hepatitis (D_3: 40 patients); and post-necrotic cirrhosis (D_4: 77 patients). The laboratory profile on which the differential diagnosis is to be made consists of four liver enzymes (U/L): aspartate aminotransferase (X_1: abbreviated *AST*); alanine aminotransferase (X_2: *ALT*); glutamate dehydrogenase (X_3: *GLDH*); and ornithine carbonyltransferase (X_4: *OCT*). The diagnosis of acute viral hepatitis was based on classical clinico-biological signs. All other patients were diagnosed on the basis of laparoscopy and biopsy findings.

In order to fulfill the normality assumptions of classical discriminant analysis, all variables were transformed by taking the natural logarithm of the observed value. The mean values and standard deviations of the four enzymes in each disease group are given in Table 5.1, together with their univariate diagnostic ability: an F-test from analysis of variance with 3 and 214 degrees of freedom. All F-values are highly significant, indicating that each enzyme discriminates among at least some of the four diseases. Using the log transform, Healy plots were calculated separately for each of the four sets of enzyme vectors. An example is given in Appendix II. All data were included in the subsequent discriminant analyses.

TABLE 5.1 Mean ± S.D. and Univariate Diagnostic Ability of Log-Enzyme Data Collected from 218 Patients with Liver Diseases

	Disease groups				Diagnostic ability
Enzyme	D_1 $n = 57$	D_2 $n = 44$	D_3 $n = 40$	D_4 $n = 77$	F-test (3 and 214 d.f.)
log(AST)	5.24 ± .67	3.79 ± .64	4.77 ± .93	4.44 ± .52	43.99
log(ALT)	6.26 ± .56	4.35 ± .69	4.82 ± .95	3.97 ± .54	136.88
log(GLDH)	2.52 ± .51	1.88 ± .44	3.03 ± .71	2.32 ± .66	27.55
log(OCT)	5.76 ± .75	4.52 ± .76	6.10 ± 1.0	5.18 ± .91	33.48

TABLE 5.2 Stepwise Variable Selection Applied to Log-Enzyme Data Collected from 218 Patients with Liver Diseases

Selection step	Enzyme selection	F-test of improvement	Degrees of freedom	Significance level
1	log(ALT)	136.88	3 and 214	$p < 0.001$
2	+ log(AST)	94.76	3 and 213	$p < 0.001$
3	+ log(GLDH)	14.31	3 and 212	$p < 0.001$
4	+ log(OCT)	0.22	3 and 211	N.S.

Source: Plomteaux (1980).

We applied multinormal discriminant analysis (Dixon and Brown, 1979) to the sample data in a stepwise manner in order to select only those variables that jointly provide a satisfactory solution to the differential diagnostic problem. As seen from Table 5.2, *AST* ($F = 94.76, p < 0.001$) and *GLDH* ($F = 14.31$, $p < 0.001$), in this order, significantly improve the diagnostic ability of *ALT*. Adding *OCT* to this triplet contributes only repetitious information ($F = 0.22$, *N.S.*)

Since there are four groups, three discriminant functions [equation (5.10)] are required, computed as:

TABLE 5.3 Classification Matrix Obtained by Reallocating 218 Patients of the Training Sample by Means of Normal Linear Discriminant Analysis Applied to the Three Selected Enzymes

	True groups			
Allocated groups	D_1	D_2	D_3	D_4
D_1	54	4	2	0
D_2	2	40	4	0
D_3	1	0	24	14
D_4	0	0	10	63
Total	57	44	40	77
Correct allocation rate (%)	94.7	90.9	60.0	81.8

$$
\begin{aligned}
l_1(\mathbf{x}) &= -8.63 \log(AST) + 13.34 \log(ALT) \\
&\quad - 1.89 \log(GLDH) - 21.60 + \log(p_1/p_4) \\
l_2(\mathbf{x}) &= -7.30 \log(AST) + 7.71 \log(ALT) \\
&\quad - 1.39 \log(GLDH) + 1.43 + \log(p_2/p_4) \\
l_3(\mathbf{x}) &= -1.79 \log(AST) + 2.80 \log(ALT) \\
&\quad + 1.49 \log(GLDH) - 7.22 + \log(p_3/p_4)
\end{aligned}
$$

Assuming that the prior probabilities were those observed in the sample, namely 0.26, 0.20, 0.18 and 0.35, all patients were reallocated using the diagnostic rule (equation 5.11). The overall classification rate was 83% (Table 5.3). Using the "leaving-one-out" (or "jackknife") method, the total correct diagnostic rate drops to 81.7%. These techniques of measuring the performance of the linear classification rule are described in greater detail at the end of this chapter (Section 5.6).

More than 90% of the cases of acute viral hepatitis and persistent chronic hepatitis and more than 80% of cirrhoses are correctly classified. The group of patients with aggressive chronic hepatitis exhibit a much larger proportion of misclassifications, since only 60% of the patients were assigned to the correct group and 25% of them are found in the cirrhosis group. Actually, aggressive chronic hepatitis and post-necrotic cirrhosis constitute two patient populations that are difficult to dissociate; this is not surprising because even histological criteria cannot always clearly distinguish these two disorders.

How would this diagnostic rule be used in practice? Consider a patient suffering from one of the diseases, but which one is unknown. Suppose that the enzyme activities recorded for him or her are $AST = 92$ U/L, $ALT = 120$ U/L, and $GLDH = 6$ U/L, respectively. First, we calculate the value of the three discriminant functions, which for this particular patient are $1_1(\mathbf{x}) = -0.14$, $1_2(\mathbf{x}) = 2.28$, and $1_3(\mathbf{x}) = 0.76$, respectively. Then, using the equation (5.9), the probabilities of belonging to each diseased group are: acute viral hepatitis (6%); persistent chronic hepatitis (71%); aggressive chronic hepatitis (16%); and cirrhosis (7%). Thus, the patient is allocated to the persistent chronic hepatitis group.

5.5 LOGISTIC DISCRIMINATION

Linear discriminant analysis based on normality assumptions provides a simple, easy-to-use method for interpreting a laboratory profile when differential diagnosis is required. Unfortunately, if it is easy to normalize a laboratory test distribution in one population, it is far more difficult to find a single transformation that can normalize the distributions of the same test in each of several diseased populations. Moreover, a profile may contain binary tests (negative/positive test) as well as continuous-valued variables. All the particular clinical situations discussed in Chapter 4 occur when more than two groups are considered. In that chapter, we postulated an exponential model for the likelihood ratio, noting that it was generally applicable to these more complex problems. We showed in Section 5.4 [equation (5.7)] that the likelihood ratios needed for discriminant analysis between g populations all followed the same exponential model. As a consequence, the predictive values as given by equation (5.9) were expressible in a simple form involving only exponential functions.

A. The Logistic Model

The logistic approach to discrimination is based on parametric assumptions about the likelihood ratios $L_{ig}(\mathbf{x})$ rather than the individual probability distribution $\mathrm{pr}(\mathbf{x}|D_i)$ of $\mathbf{X}$ in each diseased group, as in the multinormal approach.

Let $\mathbf{X}$ denote the vector of variables, no restriction being made on the nature of the variables whether discrete or continuous. We proceed under the general assumption that the likelihood ratios (5.3) have a simple exponential form,

$$L_{ig}(\mathbf{x}) = \exp(a_{0i} + \mathbf{a}_i^T\mathbf{x}) \qquad (i = 1, \ldots, g) \tag{5.14}$$

where a_{0i} denotes the intercept and $\mathbf{a}_i^T = (a_{i1}, \ldots, a_{ik})$, the vector of weights associated with the variables involved. As before, for convenience $a_{0g} = 0$ and $\mathbf{a}_g = \mathbf{0}$.

Clearly, the assumptions (5.14) hold for the multinormal model, as shown by equation (5.7). Its applicability is much wider, however. Anderson (1972) showed that the model (5.14) applies to a large family of multivariate distributions involving discrete variables, continuous variables or a mixture of both. Moreover, the continuous variables need not necessarily be normally distributed, but can be skewed in one group and fairly symmetric in another. In fact, it is now recognized that the logistic model is a satisfactory approximation to most differential diagnostic situations encountered in clinical and laboratory practice.

Under the general assumptions (5.14) for the likelihood ratios, the posterior probabilities (5.2) become

$$\mathrm{pr}(D_i|\mathbf{x}) = \frac{\exp(a_{0i}^* + \mathbf{a}_i^T\mathbf{x})}{\sum_{j=1}^{g} \exp(a_{0j}^* + \mathbf{a}_j^T\mathbf{x})} \qquad (i = 1, \ldots, g) \tag{5.15}$$

where for convenience $\overset{*}{a}_{0i} = a_{0i} + \log(p_i/p_g)$. Equations (5.15) are similar to equations (5.9), but (5.15) applies to much more general forms of **X** than just normally distributed vectors. Model (5.15) is called the "generalized logistic model" because it is the generalization of the classical logistic function

$$y(t) = \frac{\exp(t)}{1 + \exp(t)} \qquad -\infty < t < +\infty$$

to more than two groups. Finally, as in the previous section, let

$$1_i(\mathbf{x}) = a_{0i} + \log(p_i/p_g) + \mathbf{a}_i^T\mathbf{x} \qquad (i = 1, \ldots, g) \qquad (5.16)$$

denote the set of "linear logistic discriminant functions."

B. Estimating the Parameters of the Logistic Model

Under the more general assumptions (5.14), the method described in Section 5.4 (B) for estimating the a-coefficients can no longer be used, since we do not know how these are related to the parameters of the populations (e.g., $\boldsymbol{\mu}$, $\boldsymbol{\Sigma}$ in the multinormal case). Therefore, another estimation procedure has to be found. The complete solution to this problem appears in theoretical papers by Anderson (1972) and Albert and Anderson (1984). Here, we briefly outline the way to proceed.

We want to estimate the intercepts a_{0i} and the coefficient vectors $\mathbf{a}_i$ $(i = 1, \ldots, g)$, for if these are known, so are the likelihood ratios and the posterior probabilities (provided the prior probabilities are also available). In a basic paper, Anderson (1972) has shown that given a sample of n multivariate observations, n_1 belonging to disease D_1, n_2 to disease D_2 and so forth $(n = n_1 + n_2 + \cdots + n_g)$, maximum likelihood ($ML$) estimates of $\overset{*}{a}_{0i}$ and $\mathbf{a}_i$ $(i = 1, \ldots, g)$ are obtained by maximizing the function

$$\lambda = \prod_{i=1}^{g} \prod_{j=1}^{n_i} \frac{\exp(a_{0i}^* + \mathbf{a}_i^T \mathbf{x}_{ij})}{\sum_{s=1}^{g} \exp(a_{0s}^* + \mathbf{a}_s^T \mathbf{x}_{sj})} \tag{5.17}$$

with respect to the a-parameters.

Let $\hat{a}_{0i}^*$ and $\hat{\mathbf{a}}_i$ $(i = 1, \ldots, g)$ be the maximum likelihood estimates. The function (5.17) is called the likelihood function of the sample and should not be confused with the likelihood ratio function. It is important to note that the same function (5.17) is maximized whether the sample of observations is drawn from the mixture of the g populations, or whether distinct samples are taken separately from each population. The maximization of (5.17) with respect to the unknown a's is not straightforward, but iterative procedures have been developed, and the maximum is usually obtained after ten to a dozen iterations. Now, the *ML* estimates of the parameters appearing in the likelihood ratio equation (5.14) are the same as those obtained from maximizing λ in (5.17), except that the intercepts require a minor adjustment,

$$\hat{a}_{0i} = \hat{a}_{0i}^* + \log(n_g/n_i) \tag{5.18}$$

This last result is important. It was used in Chapter 4; when $g = 2$, $D_1 = D$, $D_2 = \overline{D}$, and $\hat{a} = \hat{a}^* + \log\{n(\overline{D})/n(D)\}$.

Since we have estimated the parameters involved in the likelihood ratios, these can be calculated for any future observation $\mathbf{x}$, using the equation

$$L_{ig}(\mathbf{x}) = \exp(\hat{a}_{0i} + \hat{\mathbf{a}}_i^T \mathbf{x})$$

in which the coefficients are now known. Likewise, estimated discriminant functions and posterior probabilities, respectively, are given by:

$$1_i(\mathbf{x}) = \hat{a}_{0i} + \log(p_i/p_g) + \hat{\mathbf{a}}_i^T \mathbf{x}$$

and

$$\text{pr}(D_i|\mathbf{x}) = \frac{\exp\{1_i(\mathbf{x})\}}{\sum_{j=1}^{g} \exp\{1_j(\mathbf{x})\}}$$

in which only the prior probabilities (p_i) need to be supplied. The fact that these priors can be changed independently of the a's in the last two equations gives the discrimination method its power and wide-range applicability. The logistic method provides a general solution to the problem of discriminating between a certain number of groups on the basis of a multivariate observation. We can recommend it in all instances, although when the variables are normally distributed in every group, the classical multinormal technique should be used.

C. Stepwise Variable Selection

The procedure described in Section 5.4 (C) for the multinormal model also applies to logistic discrimination, except that a chi-square test* with $g - 1$ degrees of freedom is used instead of an F-test when assessing univariate diagnostic ability and determining the subset of variables to be included in multivariate discriminant functions.

D. Medical Application: Differential Diagnosis of Liver Disease by Means of an Enzyme Profile

We applied multiple group logistic discrimination to the same data set as in Section 5.4 (D). Since this method has been

---

*If λ_k and λ_{k+1} denote the maximized likelihood function (5.17) when, respectively, k and $k + 1$ variables are considered, the criterion $2\log(\lambda_{k+1}/\lambda_k)$ is asymptotically (i.e., for large sample size n) distributed as a chi-square test with $g - 1$ degrees of freedom. When $k = 0$, then $\lambda_0 = \exp\{n_1\log(n_1/n) + \cdots + n_g\log(n_g/n)\}$.

shown to be robust and applicable to a large number of multivariate distributions, irrespective of whether the variables were discrete or continuous, no transformation was used.

The univariate diagnostic ability of each enzyme was highly significant. Using a χ^2-test on 3 degrees of freedom, we found a value of 165.27 for *ALT*, 78.84 for *AST*, 70.42 for *OCT*, and 66.43 for *GLDH*. These results agree with those found in Table 5.1 using the classical F-test on the log enzyme values.

Performing a stepwise selection of the variables, we found that only *AST* ($\chi^2 = 120.5$, 3 d.f., $p < 0.001$) and *GLDH* ($\chi^2 = 39.3$, 3 d.f., $p < 0.001$), in this order, improved the diagnostic ability of *ALT*. The addition of the variable *OCT* yielded a χ^2-value of 6.77 on 3 degrees of freedom (N.S.) and was therefore discarded from the profile. These results are in complete agreement with those found with the classical approach.

We then maximized the likelihood of the sample (5.17) by means of a computer program, derived the three logistic discriminant functions, namely,

$$\begin{aligned}
l_1(\mathbf{x}) &= -0.055\,(AST) + 0.073\,(ALT) - 0.17\,(GLDH) - 1.63 \\
&\quad + \log(p_1/p_4) \\
l_2(\mathbf{x}) &= -0.057\,(AST) + 0.063\,(ALT) - 0.24\,(GLDH) \\
&\quad + 1.70 + \log(p_2/p_4) \\
l_3(\mathbf{x}) &= -0.021\,(AST) + 0.042\,(ALT) \\
&\quad + 0.061\,(GLDH) - 2.40 + \log(p_3/p_4)
\end{aligned}$$

and obtained 83% correct diagnoses by the resubstitution method (see Section 5.6). The classification matrix is given in Table 5.4. Although the overall correct rate is the same as for the multinormal approach, the number of correctly diagnosed patients in each group is not exactly similar.

We applied the logistic diagnostic rule to the patient previously described, namely, with *AST* = 92 U/L, *ALT* = 120 U/L and *GLDH* = 6 U/L. The three discriminant functions

TABLE 5.4 Classification Matrix Obtained by Reallocating 218 Patients with Liver Diseases by Means of Logistic Discriminant Functions

Predicted diagnosis	True diagnosis			
	D_1	D_2	D_3	D_4
D_1	52	2	1	0
D_2	3	38	1	0
D_3	2	1	22	8
D_4	0	3	16	69
Total	57	44	40	77
Correction allocation rate (%)	91.2	86.4	55.0	89.6

above were calculated, assuming priors equal to the subsample proportions: $1_1(\mathbf{x}) = 0.75$, $1_2(\mathbf{x}) = 2.02$ and $1_3(\mathbf{x}) = 0.42$. The posterior probabilities for the four groups are 18%, 62%, 12% and 8%, respectively, confirming the diagnosis of persistent chronic hepatitis.

5.6 ASSESSMENT OF THE PERFORMANCE OF THE CLASSIFICATION RULE

Once the diagnostic rule has been derived, using either the multinormal or the logistic model, it is important to assess its performance in allocating patients to the various disease categories.

Let π_i ($i = 1, \ldots, g$) be the probability that a patient suffering from disease D_i will be correctly diagnosed by means of the classification rule. Likewise, denote by π the total probability of correct classification, that is the probability that a randomly selected patient will be correctly identified with respect to his or her diagnostic group. Since a priori the chances of belonging to one of the g groups are $p_1, \ldots, p_g$, respectively, the total probability of correct classification is given by

$$\pi = p_1\pi_1 + p_2\pi_2 + \cdots + p_g\pi_g = \sum_{i=1}^{g} p_i\pi_i \qquad (5.20)$$

The quantity π, or its complement $\epsilon = 1 - \pi$, the total error rate, provides an overall appraisal of the performance of the classification rule. There are several methods for estimating the probabilities π_i. We will briefly review the most common.

A. Resubstitution Method

The most familiar technique for assessing the performance of an allocation rule is called the resubstitution method. We already referred to it in the previous example. It consists of re-allocating all patients of the training sample by means of the estimated classification rule and matching predicted versus actual diagnosis. Let r_i be the number of patients correctly allocated to D_i. We estimate π_i by

$$\hat{\pi}_i = \frac{r_i}{n_i} \qquad (i = 1, \ldots, g) \qquad (5.21)$$

Assuming $p_1, \ldots, p_g$ are known or estimated separately,

$$\hat{\pi} = \sum_{i=1}^{g} p_i \frac{r_i}{n_i} \qquad (5.22)$$

Note that if the sample of size n is drawn randomly from the mixture of the diseased categories, $\hat{p}_i = n_i/n$, and

$$\hat{\pi} = \sum_{i=1}^{g} \frac{n_i}{n}\frac{r_i}{n_i} = \frac{1}{n}\sum_{i=1}^{g} r_i$$

The resubstitution method, because it uses the same sample data to derive the classification rule and to assess its performance, leads to an overestimation of the diagnostic performance of the rule, that is, overestimates of π_i and π.

B. The "Leaving-One-Out," or "Jackknife," Method

This method was proposed by Lachenbruch (1967) for obtaining more realistic estimates of π_i. It proceeds as follows:

1. Take one patient out of the total sample of n patients.
2. Derive the classification rule from this reduced sample of $n - 1$ observations.
3. Allocate the dropped-out patient by means of the classification rule obtained in step 2. If the patient is correctly allocated to the appropriate disease group D_i, add 1 to the number of patients correctly classified to this group (r_i').
4. Repeat steps 1 to 3 for all patients of the sample.
5. Estimate the quantities π_i by

$$\hat{\pi}_i^* = \frac{r_i'}{n_i} \qquad (i = 1, \ldots, g)$$
$$\hat{\pi}^* = \sum_{i=1}^{g} p_i \frac{r_i'}{n_i} \tag{5.23}$$

It can be proven that the number r_i' of correctly allocated subjects to group D_i by means of the leaving-one-out method is always less than or equal to the number r_i of correctly allocated patients for group D_i by means of the resubstitution method, whence

$$\hat{\pi}_i^* \leq \hat{\pi}_i \qquad \text{and} \qquad \hat{\pi}^* \leq \hat{\pi}$$

The leaving-one-out procedure can consume a great deal of computer time since it requires the calculation of n classification rules, one for each patient left out. When the multinormal model is used to derive the classification rule, the resubstitution and leaving-one-out methods can be performed simultaneously. However, this is not true under logistic discrimination, which requires an iterative estimation procedure each time. So in this case, the leaving-one-out technique is not really appropriate, and other means must be looked for to overcome the weakness of the resubstitution method.

C. The Validation Sample Method

Ideally, the classification rule derived from one sample of patients should be applied to an independent set of data, a so-called validation sample. Although not always feasible, the validation sample method is probably the best way to measure how well a diagnostic rule works in practice. Sometimes the original sample of data is sufficiently large to be split into two sets, one for estimation and the other for validation.

Appendix I: Liver Enzyme Data

GROUP 1 Acute Viral Hepatitis

Patient	Group	AST	ALT	GLDH	OCT
1	1	236	582	10	457
2	1	65	258	20	242
3	1	59	244	16	236
4	1	92	120	6	205
5	1	99	352	13	315
6	1	87	380	7	92
7	1	202	429	15	715
8	1	208	539	14	480
9	1	105	465	4	58
10	1	95	442	13	229
11	1	215	570	17	360
12	1	101	277	6	124
13	1	454	639	27	712
14	1	308	1243	9	470
15	1	82	294	11	236
16	1	196	760	18	249
17	1	141	550	24	610
18	1	73	201	3	66
19	1	569	1354	24	996
20	1	125	390	10	315
21	1	77	480	9	231

GROUP 1 Acute Viral Hepatitis (*continued*)

Patient	Group	AST	ALT	GLDH	OCT
22	1	78	495	12	299
23	1	165	330	21	402
24	1	214	680	10	266
25	1	141	539	21	326
26	1	220	990	18	321
27	1	127	480	18	630
28	1	324	936	2	316
29	1	149	334	13	370
30	1	270	465	10	347
31	1	178	660	12	336
32	1	202	693	19	607
33	1	56	158	6	116
34	1	129	704	14	225
35	1	682	1595	20	960
36	1	290	987	20	202
37	1	61	327	14	281
38	1	289	693	9	556
39	1	133	470	11	363
40	1	170	620	13	318
41	1	550	1034	18	995
42	1	313	414	13	870
43	1	166	239	10	288
44	1	340	840	12	680
45	1	660	1287	21	4100
46	1	321	1254	18	965
47	1	401	492	22	596
48	1	665	970	14	1040
49	1	242	528	16	847
50	1	339	627	11	603
51	1	372	910	19	368
52	1	165	584	9	413
53	1	385	610	13	512
54	1	152	270	7	152
55	1	605	1199	16	1628
56	1	247	452	23	720
57	1	123	231	11	323

GROUP 2 Persistent Chronic Hepatitis

Patient	Group	AST	ALT	GLDH	OCT
1	2	473	506	13	960
2	2	40	52	5	79

GROUP 2 Persistent Chronic Hepatitis (*continued*)

Patient	Group	AST	ALT	GLDH	OCT
3	2	53	123	7	201
4	2	76	133	8	158
5	2	31	63	4	126
6	2	32	56	6	35
7	2	50	59	9	63
8	2	56	72	7	57
9	2	39	87	9	95
10	2	46	95	8	111
11	2	29	57	5	65
12	2	40	50	3	51
13	2	29	44	4	28
14	2	77	132	7	130
15	2	28	44	4	57
16	2	28	68	5	41
17	2	34	58	6	66
18	2	24	42	3	35
19	2	34	61	7	165
20	2	119	345	23	202
21	2	26	41	5	54
22	2	39	84	5	55
23	2	30	70	7	209
24	2	35	81	8	79
25	2	29	41	7	39
26	2	31	38	5	25
27	2	31	56	6	74
28	2	23	43	7	72
29	2	38	40	6	57
30	2	22	42	4	39
31	2	26	57	7	85
32	2	26	42	17	231
33	2	35	72	3	35
34	2	42	53	7	147
35	2	41	47	10	190
36	2	64	260	5	180
37	2	212	660	14	321
38	2	83	101	5	195
39	2	64	185	10	231
40	2	121	159	9	179
41	2	29	42	4	30
42	2	129	163	9	140
43	2	76	109	10	180
44	2	20	57	7	72

GROUP 3 Aggressive Chronic Hepatitis

Patient	Group	AST	ALT	GLDH	OCT
1	3	135	118	50	1023
2	3	75	125	19	969
3	3	120	163	16	396
4	3	99	224	21	294
5	3	112	93	52	1104
6	3	71	61	6	84
7	3	144	42	6	147
8	3	52	86	19	214
9	3	46	40	9	117
10	3	49	51	13	198
11	3	266	316	23	364
12	3	52	30	19	129
13	3	139	132	47	2100
14	3	50	89	15	162
15	3	53	31	4	51
16	3	216	146	24	399
17	3	246	114	24	612
18	3	74	115	24	513
19	3	137	94	18	438
20	3	70	53	8	333
21	3	80	55	8	162
22	3	115	58	13	381
23	3	119	132	9	249
24	3	222	204	15	279
25	3	660	418	28	1515
26	3	159	197	23	699
27	3	86	52	18	687
28	3	103	118	17	204
29	3	91	52	27	513
30	3	110	32	18	294
31	3	192	255	25	528
32	3	540	184	160	5067
33	3	490	425	41	534
34	3	2298	1310	43	4928
35	3	858	1551	29	2487
36	3	87	139	34	585
37	3	184	112	28	192
38	3	100	94	52	696
39	3	1561	979	31	630
40	3	276	209	39	1041

GROUP 4 Post-necrotic Cirrhosis

Patient	Group	AST	ALT	GLDH	OCT
1	4	173	121	34	1005
2	4	42	24	4	51
3	4	44	28	15	210
4	4	83	67	3	66
5	4	86	59	11	297
6	4	42	25	3	21
7	4	45	26	3	18
8	4	76	54	13	255
9	4	704	172	75	420
10	4	91	64	9	159
11	4	106	61	12	171
12	4	127	62	16	291
13	4	101	57	7	103
14	4	71	51	6	189
15	4	93	78	21	312
16	4	76	69	10	228
17	4	110	79	8	204
18	4	82	55	6	65
19	4	57	37	5	54
20	4	72	31	7	120
21	4	62	26	11	162
22	4	143	104	8	189
23	4	80	51	6	78
24	4	207	83	5	147
25	4	84	54	6	105
26	4	132	72	11	237
27	4	80	50	10	525
28	4	118	84	14	207
29	4	42	22	4	66
30	4	47	26	7	75
31	4	108	59	24	273
32	4	70	65	9	669
33	4	41	34	7	105
34	4	53	31	6	54
35	4	107	175	20	228
36	4	140	68	15	375
37	4	121	74	9	369
38	4	63	36	50	750
39	4	80	85	12	204
40	4	325	141	31	2010

GROUP 4 Post-necrotic Cirrhosis (*continued*)

Patient	Group	AST	ALT	GLDH	OCT
41	4	43	19	5	51
42	4	47	29	8	36
43	4	135	90	46	1161
44	4	187	163	15	501
45	4	142	74	11	228
46	4	48	23	6	138
47	4	119	62	18	288
48	4	56	18	10	186
49	4	53	39	13	222
50	4	121	79	7	184
51	4	54	52	25	324
52	4	99	45	11	222
53	4	114	74	14	264
54	4	61	32	7	147
55	4	71	52	9	144
56	4	54	34	5	40
57	4	43	37	12	120
58	4	52	45	7	159
59	4	91	43	4	93
60	4	43	22	7	48
61	4	119	73	21	504
62	4	115	89	9	204
63	4	55	34	5	51
64	4	141	78	53	924
65	4	63	38	11	249
66	4	40	30	6	54
67	4	78	32	17	270
68	4	175	134	21	516
69	4	132	69	9	174
70	4	142	93	10	258
71	4	71	42	9	225
72	4	67	44	17	276
73	4	168	154	14	384
74	4	89	63	10	426
75	4	101	76	6	99
76	4	82	49	6	102
77	4	63	46	10	81

Source: Reproduced by permission of G. Plomteux, Ph.D.

APPENDIX II: HEALY PLOT, AN EXAMPLE

Figure 5.3 illustrates a Healy plot for detecting outliers among a set of multivariate vectors. Using the natural logarithms of the observations, values of $D^2(\mathbf{x}_0) = (\mathbf{x}_0 - \overline{\mathbf{x}})^T \mathbf{S}^{-1} (\mathbf{x}_0 - \overline{\mathbf{x}})$ (see Chapter 3, p. 60; also referred to as $\hat{Q}$ in Chapter 2, Section 2.5) were computed for the observed vectors of four liver enzymes in 57 patients with acute viral hepatitis (Appendix I, Group 1). The graph of $\sqrt{D^2}$ on normal probability paper shows a break at $\sqrt{D^2} > 2.5$. However, the six $\sqrt{D^2}$ values beyond this point show approximately the same slope as the 33 values less than 2.0. This seemed good reason not to exclude any of these profiles from the discriminant function analysis. This

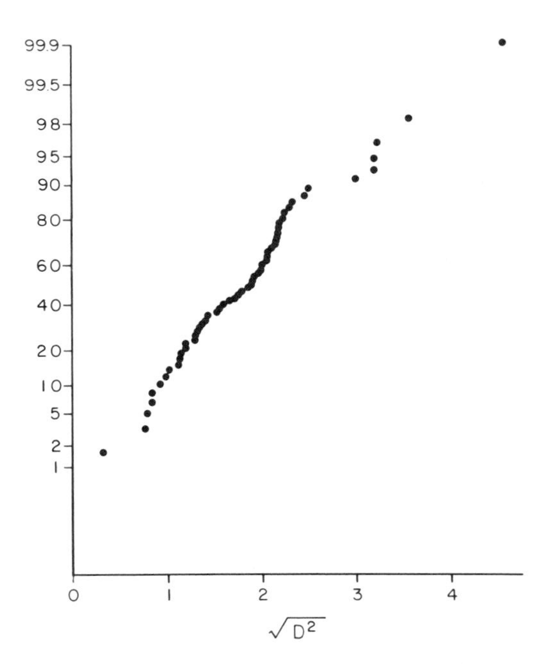

FIGURE 5.3 Normal probability plots of $\sqrt{D^2}$ for the joint distribution of the logs of four liver enzymes in 57 patients with acute viral hepatitis.

judgment was confirmed by a nonsignificant Kolmogorov-Smirnov test for multivariate normality applied to all 57 vectors.

Similar results were found for the data from each of the other three groups with liver diseases discussed in this chapter, except for one patient profile: Patient No. 9 in Group 4, post-necrotic cirrhosis (see Appendix I). This patient's enzyme vector, after transforming to logs, yielded a $\sqrt{D^2}$ value of 6.16. However, with no other apparent reason (e.g., laboratory error) for excluding this profile, the decision was made to keep it in the dataset.

REFERENCES

Albert, A. and Anderson, J. A. (1984): On the existence of maximum likelihood estimates in logistic regression models. *Biometrika 71*, 1–10.

Anderson, J. A. (1972): Separate sample logistic discrimination. *Biometrika 59*, 19–35.

Anderson, T. W. (1958): *An Introduction to Multivariate Statistical Analysis.* Wiley, New York, pp. 133 et seq.

Cacoullos, T. (1973): *Discriminant Analysis and Applications.* Academic Press, New York.

Dixon, W. J. and Brown, M. B. (1979): *Biomedical Computer Programs P-Series (BMDP 7M).* University of California Press, Berkeley, Ca.

Fukunaga, K. (1972): *Introduction to Statistical Pattern Recognition.* Academic Press, New York.

Lachenbruch, P. A. (1967): An almost unbiased method for obtaining confidence intervals for the probability of misclassification in discriminant analysis. *Biometrics 23*, 639–645.

Lachenbruch, P. A. (1975): *Discriminant Analysis.* Hafner Press, New York.

Plomteux, G. (1980): Multivariate analysis of an enzyme profile for the differential diagnosis of viral hepatitis. *Clin. Chem. 26*, 1897–1899.

Solberg, H. E. (1978): Discriminant analysis. *CRC Crit. Rev. Clin Lab. Sci. 9*, 209–242.

6

PROGNOSIS

6.1
PROBLEM FORMULATION

In Chapters 4 and 5, we discussed statistical aspects of differential diagnosis and described methods for allocating patients to one of several disease categories on the basis of a laboratory profile. There is another important area in which laboratory determinations can help the physician's daily decisions, namely medical prognosis. Prognosis is the process of predicting the future medical condition of a patient, based in part on information about the patient's present condition. Most often, the physician is interested in predicting the outcome of a particular disease. The outcome variable may be binary: death or survival; remission or nonremission; complications or no complications; favorable or unfavorable evolution. Sometimes more than two possibilities are defined. For example, in neurosurgery, the Glasgow Outcome Scale (Jennett and Bond, 1975) considers consequences of severe head injury: good recovery, moderate disability, severe disability, permanent vegetative state, and death.

Denote by $\mathbf{X}^T = (X_1, \ldots, X_k)$ a vector of laboratory tests and other relevant numerical descriptors of the patient. Let $O_1, \ldots, O_g$ represent g outcome categories. One statistical problem consists of calculating for a given $\mathbf{x}$ the posterior probability of each outcome, $\text{pr}(O_i|\mathbf{x})$. This problem looks similar to that discussed in Chapter 5, and it is indeed. However, from the statistical point of view, major differences exist between the two situations. Most importantly, differential diagnosis is generally concerned with "qualitatively" distinct disease groups. That is, the diseases $D_1, \ldots, D_g$ are not usually ordered in any obvious way. In contrast, the outcome categories $O_1, \ldots, O_g$ in a prognostic problem, while they may certainly differ in the quality of life involved, are also "quantitative" in the sense that they may be arranged in order of increasing or decreasing severity. Thus, under the Glasgow scale, if O_1 represents good recovery and O_3 severe disability, we would not use O_2 to represent death. That outcome would be labeled O_5.

From a mathematical point of view, this distinction between diagnostic and prognostic situations may be formalized by introducing a new variable Y that defines the group categories. Specifically, if E denotes the set of values taken by the variable Y, a patient belongs to group D_i (or outcome O_i) if and only if $y \in E_i$, where the sets $E_1, \ldots, E_g$ form a partition of E. In the case of differential diagnosis, Y is simply a dummy variable identifying the g groups. That is, $E = \{1, \ldots, g\}$ and $E_i = \{i\}$, $(i = 1, \ldots, g)$. In the prognostic situation, on the other hand, Y becomes a continuous-valued variable whose value for a given patient defines what might be called the risk status of that patient. Thus, a patient belongs to outcome group O_i if and only if $\theta_{i-1} < y \leq \theta_i$, where the constants θ_i $(i = 1, \ldots, g)$ are threshold levels on the y scale, and, by convention, $\theta_0 = -\infty$, $\theta_g = +\infty$. The range of Y is then the real line ($E = R$) and $E_i = [\theta_{i-1}, \theta_i]$. Although the precise value y is indeterminate, the practical problem consists of predicting in which set (E_i) y lies, given the profile $\mathbf{x}$, for this determines the predicted outcome.

When dealing with prognosis, it is important to state clearly the period in which the outcomes occur. For instance, with a patient who has suffered a heart attack and been admitted to the coronary care unit, one may be interested in only death or survival while the patient is still under intensive care. Alternatively, survival or nonsurvival up to hospital discharge may be the chief concern, or the time period of surveillance may be extended to one year after discharge. These examples correspond to short-, middle-, and long-term predictions, and the laboratory tests used to make these predictions may be quite different. The inflammation marker α_1-acid glycoprotein is useless for short-term prognosis but very helpful for long-term risk assessments (Chapelle et al., 1983).

Finally, data involved in an acute prognostic problem are likely to be of a serial nature, for example, repeated daily when day-to-day reassessment of risk and prediction of outcome are desired. Such serial measurements form short time series with both random and deterministic elements. They require special statistical treatment. Such methods will be discussed in Chapter 7.

6.2 TWO-OUTCOME PREDICTION PROBLEM: THE LOGISTIC MODEL

The most familiar prognostic situation involves only two outcomes, e.g., survival–death, remission–nonremission. Given a patient suffering from disease D, the statistical problem consists of predicting his or her outcome O_1 or O_2, on the basis of some vector $\mathbf{X}$ of laboratory tests and clinical data. We need to calculate the probability of each outcome, $\text{pr}(O_1|\mathbf{x})$ and $\text{pr}(O_2|\mathbf{x})$.

Now this can be thought of simply as a discrimination problem, as discussed in Chapters 4 and 5, so that the methods developed for diagnosis apply equally well here. For instance, the application of logistic discriminant analysis yields a linear combination of the variables

$$I = a_0 + a_1x_1 + \cdots + a_kx_k \tag{6.1}$$

and the probability of an unfavorable outcome O_2 would be calculated from the logistic equation

$$\text{pr}(O_2|\mathbf{x}) = \frac{\exp(I)}{1 + \exp(I)} \tag{6.2}$$

The probability of a favorable outcome O_1 is given by $1 - \text{pr}(O_2|\mathbf{x})$.

When dealing with prognostic situations, the discriminant function $I = a_0 + \mathbf{a}^T\mathbf{x}$ in equation (6.1) is preferably called a "risk index" or "prognostic index," because it allows both the assessment of the patient's condition and the forecast of his or her outcome. Positive values of I are a sign of poor prognosis, while negative scores correspond to lower risk patients. A value $I = 0$ means a 50% chance for each outcome. The quality of the prognostic index can be tested by comparing predicted outcomes with actual outcomes and recording the total rate of correct predictions.

Estimates of the coefficients of the risk index are obtained by maximizing the likelihood of the sample of observations as described in Chapter 5. Likewise, it is possible to select among the k variables only those that jointly provide the best prognostic information.

Example: Acute Myocardial Infarction

A random sample of 159 patients with documented acute myocardial infarction and admitted to the coronary care unit was available for defining an index to predict outcome within the first two weeks of hospitalization (Chapelle et al., 1981). Seventeen patients died within this period and 142 survived.

Three variables were studied:

1. Age in years of the patient at admission
2. Number of previous myocardial infarctions ($nMI = 0, 1, 2, \ldots$)
3. Serum activity in U/L of lactate dehydrogenase (LD) 24 hours after admission

The application of logistic discriminant analysis yielded the following risk index:

$$I = 0.0978 \text{ Age} + 1.37\, nMI + 0.00189\, LD - 11.9 \qquad (6.3)$$

One hundred and forty survivors (98.6%) and six nonsurvivors (35.3%) were predicted correctly. Assuming a prior probability of death equal to 17/159, or 10.7%, the predictive value of a positive index, i.e., pr(Death$|I > 0$), is 75% [equation (4.3)], and the predictive value of a negative index, pr(Survival$|I < 0$) is 93% [equation (4.4)]. The use of equations (6.3) and (6.2) enables us to estimate for each patient the relative risks of survival and death. Assume that a patient with acute myocardial infarction, aged 60 years, with two previous infarcts ($nMI = 2$), presents, 24 hours after admission, an LD activity of 2500 U/L. From equation (6.3), his risk score is equal to

$$I = 0.0978 \times 60 + 1.37 \times 2 + 0.00189 \times 2500 - 11.9 = 1.43$$

Thus, from equation (6.2), pr(Death$|I$) $=$ 0.81 and pr(Survival$|I$) $=$ 0.19, so that the relative risk is 4.2. The prior odds for dying are about 1:10, but a posteriori, for this particular patient, they are 4:1 indicating that he is at very high risk.

6.3 TWO-OUTCOME PREDICTION PROBLEM: THE PROBIT APPROACH

In the preceding section, we applied logistic discriminant analysis as if the problem were one of differential diagnosis, that is, as if the two outcome categories were qualitatively distinct. In fact, of course, there is an obvious ordering on the severity scale and, presumably, a threshold value θ, such that if $y \leq \theta$, outcome O_1 (survival) occurs, but if $y > \theta$, outcome O_2 occurs. The probit model*, a classical approach to the analysis of biological assays (e.g, Finney, 1971), is based explicitly on the concept of a risk status Y and threshold θ.

*The word "probit" stands for "probability unit," originally proposed by the late biometrician C. I. Bliss in the context of biological assay to denote a standard normal deviate plus 5 to eliminate negative results.

A. The Multinormal Model

When the profile $\mathbf{X}$ contains only real-valued, normally distributed variables, we can assume that the joint distribution of Y, the unobservable underlying variable, and $\mathbf{X}$ is multinormal with mean $\boldsymbol{\upsilon}$ and covariance matrix $\mathbf{V}$, where

$$\boldsymbol{\upsilon}^T = (0, \boldsymbol{\mu}^T)$$

and (6.4)

$$\mathbf{V} = \begin{bmatrix} 1 & \boldsymbol{\sigma}^T \\ \boldsymbol{\sigma} & \boldsymbol{\Sigma} \end{bmatrix}$$

As before, $\boldsymbol{\mu}$ and $\boldsymbol{\Sigma}$ represent the mean and covariance matrix of $\mathbf{X}$, respectively, while $\boldsymbol{\sigma}$ is the vector of covariances between Y and the variables of $\mathbf{X}$. Without loss of generality, we have taken the distribution of y to be a standard normal: mean zero, standard deviation unity. Under these conditions, it is easily shown that the conditional probability of outcome O_2 is given by

$$\text{pr}(O_2|\mathbf{x}) = \text{pr}(Y > \theta|\mathbf{x}) = \Phi(a_0 + \mathbf{a}^T\mathbf{x}) \quad (6.5)$$

where $\Phi(.)$, is the cumulative standard normal distribution (see Chapter 2),

$$a_0 = \frac{-(\boldsymbol{\theta} - \boldsymbol{\sigma}^T\boldsymbol{\Sigma}^{-1}\boldsymbol{\mu})}{\sqrt{1 - R^2}}$$

$$\mathbf{a}^T = \frac{\boldsymbol{\sigma}^T\boldsymbol{\Sigma}^{-1}}{\sqrt{1 - R^2}} \quad (6.6)$$

and $R = \sqrt{\boldsymbol{\sigma}^{\mathrm{T}}\boldsymbol{\Sigma}\boldsymbol{\sigma}}$, the multiple correlation coefficient between Y and $\mathbf{X}$.

Equation (6.5) shows that with the multinormal model, there is a simple relationship between the probability of outcome and the probit risk index $a_0 + \mathbf{a}^T\mathbf{x}$. When we know the value of this index, the corresponding outcome probability may be found from a standard normal distribution table.

B. A More General Model

The multinormal assumptions underlying the probit risk index prohibit our including binary or non-normally distributed variables in the observed profile. However, Albert and Anderson (1981) have shown that under the weaker assumption that the conditional distribution of Y given any $\mathbf{x}$ is univariate normal (with mean, say, $b_0 + \mathbf{b}^T\mathbf{x}$ and variance τ^2), the probit model (6.5) still holds. In other words, probit risk indices can be used for predicting outcome regardless of the nature of the k-dimensional vector $\mathbf{X}$. To illustrate, suppose we apply probit discriminant analysis to the sample of 159 patients with documented myocardial infarction described in Section 6.2. The following results (see Albert et al., 1981) were obtained by maximizing with respect to a_0 and $\mathbf{a}$ the log-likelihood of the sample

$$\log L(a_0,\mathbf{a}) = \sum_{i=1}^{159} [(1 - z_i)\log\{1 - \Phi(a_0 + \mathbf{a}^T\mathbf{x}_i)\} + z_i \log\Phi(a_0 + \mathbf{a}^T\mathbf{x}_i)]$$

where $z_i = 0$ if the ith patient survived and $z_i = 1$ if he or she died, and $\mathbf{x}_i =$ the associated values of age, nMI and LD.

The probit prognostic index was

$$I = 0.054 \text{ Age} + 0.68\, nMI + 0.000978 \text{ LD} - 6.39 \qquad (6.7)$$

Again, 140 survivors and 6 deceased were predicted correctly; this index showed exactly the same efficiency as the logistic. The probability of death for the same 60-year-old patient, with two previous myocardial infarcts ($nMI = 2$) and an LD activity of 2500 U/L 24 hours after admission, can now be obtained using equations (6.7) and (6.5):

$$I = 0.054 \times 60 + 0.68 \times 2 + 0.000978 \times 2500 - 6.39 = 0.66$$

and

$$\text{pr}(\text{Death}|I) = \Phi(0.66) = 0.75$$

This posterior probability is slightly less than that obtained using the logistic model (0.75 versus 0.81). The posterior odds for death in this case are 3:1 rather than 4:1.

We can proceed further without loss of generality to set $b_0 = 0$ and $\tau^2 = 1$ in the conditional distribution $\text{pr}(y|\mathbf{x})$. Then $\theta = -a_0$* and equation (6.7) can be interpreted in a slightly different way. We can now explicitly define the conditional mean of $Y|\mathbf{x}$ as

$$\text{Estimated } E(Y|\mathbf{x}) = 0.054 \text{ Age} + 0.68\ nMI + 0.000978\ LD$$

with threshold $\theta = 6.39$. Thus, a patient is considered at high risk if his or her estimated value of $E(Y|\mathbf{x})$ exceeds 6.39, otherwise at lower risk.

Comparing the estimated coefficients of the logistic risk index (6.3) with those of the probit index (6.7), we find that their average ratio is almost constant: 1.91 ± 0.09. This reflects the fact that the logistic and probit functions are very similar to each other. In fact, the approximation $\phi(x) = \exp(mx)/\{1 + \exp(mx)\}$, where $m = (8/\pi)^{1/2} = 1.6$, has a maximum absolute error of less than 0.02. In practice, the logistic model

---

*Since for the general probit model $a_0 = (b_0 - \theta)/\tau$ and $\mathbf{a} = \mathbf{b}/\tau$, by setting $b_0 = 0$ and $\tau^2 = 1$, $a_0 = -\theta$ and $\mathbf{a} = \mathbf{b}$. This simply corresponds to changing the zero and scale of Y.

may be preferred because it is available on any pocket or desktop calculator, whereas the cumulative standard normal distribution is not. However, if the user prefers the probit approach, the approximation mentioned above may be useful.

6.4 SEVERAL OUTCOME CATEGORIES

So far, outcome has been considered as a dichotomous response variable (e.g., survival or death). One may often wish to classify patients into several categories, placing more than one threshold point on the Y-scale. For example, when looking at the quality of recovery from an acute illness, two classes are generally not sufficient to enumerate the various possibilities. We mentioned previously the five possible consequences after severe head injury, as codified by the Glasgow Outcome Scale.

Let $O_1, \ldots, O_g$ be the g outcomes that can result in patients suffering from disease D. The outcome categories are ordered, $O_1 < O_2 < \cdots < O_g$, in the sense that O_1 is less severe than O_2, which is less severe than O_3, etc.

Again, we imagine the existence of an underlying but unobservable variable Y and a set of $g-1$ thresholds $\theta_1 < \cdots < \theta_{g-1}$ such that outcome O_1 occurs to patients for whom $y \le \theta_1$, O_2 to patients with $\theta_1 < y \le \theta_2, \ldots, O_g$ to patients with $\theta_{g-1} < y$.

In general [see Figure (6.1)],

$$\text{Outcome } O_i = \{y\colon \theta_{i-1} < y \le \theta_i\} \qquad (i = 1, \ldots, g) \qquad (6.8)$$

with the convention that $\theta_0 = -\infty$ and $\theta_g = +\infty$.

To solve the prognostic problem, we could apply the discriminant analysis described in Chapter 5 [e.g., equation (5.15)], but this is not the best way to proceed. Recall that, when discriminating among g groups, $g-1$ discriminant func-

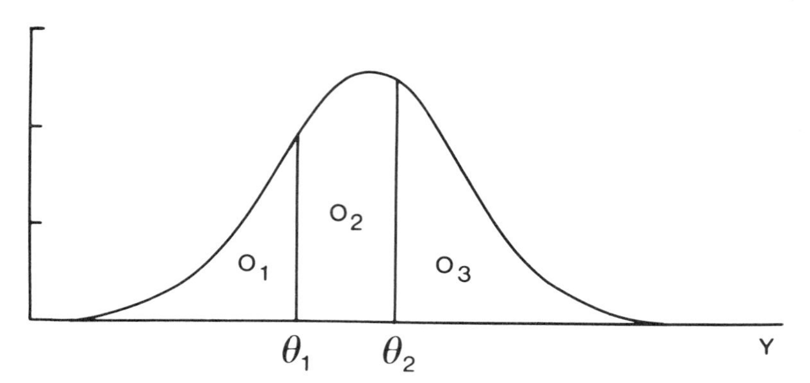

FIGURE 6.1 Definition of ordered outcome categories by means of thresholds on the scale of underlying variable Y ($g = 3$).

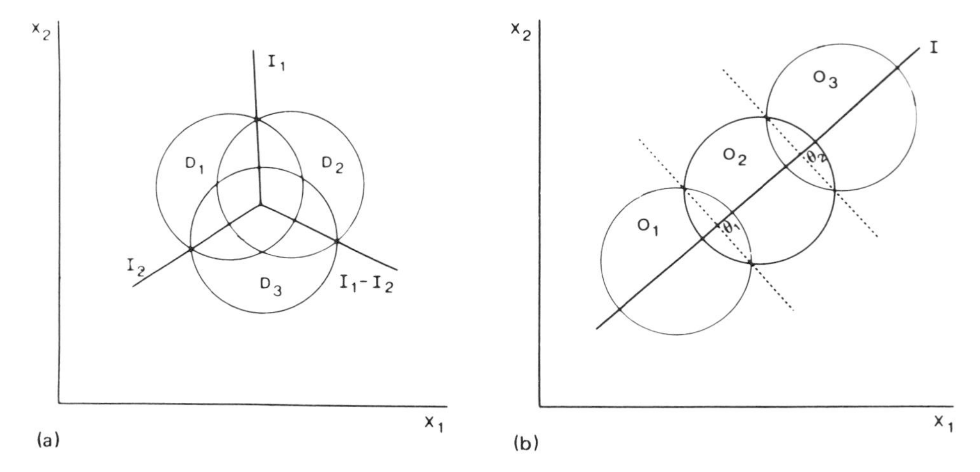

FIGURE 6.2 Discrimination between qualitatively distinct disease groups (a) and quantitatively distinct (ordered) outcome categories (b).

tions are needed to achieve a satisfactory classification. In general, the weight (coefficient) associated with a given variable X_i is different for each discriminant function, reflecting the fact that the groups occupy distinct positions in the observation space. Ordered groups, on the other hand, can be regarded as aligned clusters, so that the $g-1$ discriminant functions are all parallel. Then, the weights of each variable X_i are the same on all functions, and only the intercepts differ. The distinction between the two situations is shown in Figure 6.2 ($g = 3$).

To allocate patients into disease D_1, D_2, or D_3, we need to know the discriminant functions I_1 and I_2, since the separation between D_2 and D_3 is given by $I_1 - I_2$. In contrast, for the three outcomes O_1, O_2, or O_3, only the risk index I and the cutoff points θ_1 and θ_2 are required. We outline below the method used to estimate these quantities under the logistic model. To illustrate, three ordered outcome situations are considered.

A. Using the Logistic Model to Estimate the Parameters for Three Outcome Categories

If we assume, as in Section 6.3(B) that the conditional distribution of $Y|\mathbf{x}$ is univariate normal with mean $\mathbf{a}^T\mathbf{x}$ and variance unity, the outcome probabilities are given by the equations

$$\begin{aligned}
\text{pr}(O_1|\mathbf{x}) &= \text{pr}(y \leq \theta_1|\mathbf{x}) \\
&= \Phi(\theta_1 - \mathbf{a}^T\mathbf{x}) \\
\text{pr}(O_2|\mathbf{x}) &= \text{pr}(\theta_1 < y \leq \theta_2|\mathbf{x}) \\
&= \Phi(\theta_2 - \mathbf{a}^T\mathbf{x}) - \Phi(\theta_1 - \mathbf{a}^T\mathbf{x}) \\
\text{pr}(O_3|\mathbf{x}) &= \text{pr}(y > \theta_2|\mathbf{x}) \\
&= 1 - \Phi(\theta_2 - \mathbf{a}^T\mathbf{x})
\end{aligned} \tag{6.9}$$

These equations result immediately from the normality assumptions. They involve θ_1 and θ_2, the two thresholds, and the linear combination $I = \mathbf{a}^T\mathbf{x} = a_1x_1 + \cdots + a_kx_k$, which is the probit risk index already defined.

We mentioned previously the relationship between the probit and logistic functions, and that the latter was simpler to apply. Thus, assuming the logistic rather than the normal form for the distribution of Y given $\mathbf{x}$, equations (6.9) are replaced by

$$\begin{aligned} \mathrm{pr}(O_1|\mathbf{x}) &= \Lambda(\theta_1 - I) \\ \mathrm{pr}(O_2|\mathbf{x}) &= \Lambda(\theta_2 - I) - \Lambda(\theta_1 - I) \\ \mathrm{pr}(O_3|\mathbf{x}) &= 1 - \Lambda(\theta_2 - I) \end{aligned} \tag{6.10}$$

where $\Lambda(.) = \exp(.)/\{1 + \exp(.)\}$, and I is now the logistic index of risk. This model (Anderson and Philips, 1981) involves k + 2 parameters (θ_1, θ_2, a_1, . . . , a_k), whereas the model for three qualitatively distinct groups would contain $2(k + 1)$ parameters, substantially more.

Given a random sample of size n from a population of patients with disease D, we obtain maximum likelihood estimates of these parameters by maximizing the function

$$\log L(\theta_1,\theta_2,\mathbf{a}) = \sum_{i=1}^{n} \log \mathrm{pr}(\mathrm{Outcome}|\mathbf{x}_i) \tag{6.11}$$

where for pr(Outcome$|\mathbf{x}_i$) we substitute the appropriate equation in the set (6.10). No analytic solution exists, so that an iterative procedure must be used to obtain the estimates. From these estimates, the risk index I may be calculated and the outcome predicted for each patient. Predicted and actual outcomes are compared, and the number of correct predictions serves to test the performance of the prognostic index. The "leaving-one-out" and validation sample methods may be used to secure more realistic measures of the index's predictive ability.

TABLE 6.1 Mean Values and Standard Deviations of Age and CSF CK-BB Activity in Three Groups of Severely Head-Injured Patients

	Outcome		
	Favorable evolution $n = 19$	Unfavorable evolution $n = 8$	Death $n = 33$
Variables			
Age (years)	18 ± 12	24 ± 18	29 ± 16
CK-BB (U/L)	118 ± 91	263 ± 188	467 ± 397

B. Example: Outcome after Severe Head Injury

Sixty patients with severe head injury were admitted to the university hospital at Liège, Belgium and then classified according to the Glasgow Outcome Scale (Hans et al., 1985). Six months later, 19 had had a favorable evolution (outcome O_1), 8 were in persistent vegetative state or had severe disability (outcome O_2), and 33 had died (O_3). The age of each patient had been recorded on admission and cerebrospinal fluid CK-BB isoenzyme (U/L) was measured within the first 24 hours. The data are listed in Appendix II. Mean values and standard deviations are given in Table 6.1.

Applying the logistic model (6.10) to these two variables led to the estimated risk index,

$$I = 0.050 \text{ age} + 0.006014 \text{ CK-BB}$$

Standard errors of the coefficients were 0.021 and 0.001861, respectively. Therefore, using a standard normal deviate test, both variables may be considered significant risk factors. The estimated thresholds were $\hat{\theta}_1 = 1.78$ (± 0.67) and $\hat{\theta}_2 = 2.63$ (± 0.72), respectively, also significantly different from zero.

Calculating the index I for each of the 60 patients and allocating each to one of the three outcome categories in

TABLE 6.2 Matrix of Predicted Versus True Outcome for the Sample of 60 Patients with Severe Head Injury[a]

	True outcome		
	Favorable evolution	Unfavorable evolution	Death
Predicted outcome			
Favorable ($I \leq 1.78$)	11	2	5
Unfavorable ($1.78 < I \leq 2.63$)	7	2	5
Death ($I > 2.63$)	1	4	23
	19	8	33

[a]The risk index is given by the equation $I = 0.05$ Age $+ 0.006014$ CK-BB.

accordance with the I-value relative to $\hat{\theta}_1$ and $\hat{\theta}_2$, the statistics shown in Table 6.2 were obtained. The overall proportion of correctly predicted outcomes was 60% (36/60); 70% of the deaths were correctly predicted, as were 58% of the favorable outcomes. Prognosis was more hazardous in the intermediate group of patients who were left either in a persistent vegetative state or with severe disability. Other risk factors will have to be looked for to improve prediction within this class.

Using equations (6.10), it is possible to assess the patient's individual chances of each outcome category. Note that from the sample data, the prior probabilities of the three risk classes (O_1, O_2, O_3) are 32%, 13%, and 55%, respectively. Consider a male patient aged 29 with a CSF CK-BB activity of 80 U/L. His risk index will be

$$I = 0.050 \times 29 + 0.006014 \times 80 = 1.93$$

Clearly, I falls between the two cutoff points $\hat{\theta}_1 = 1.78$ and $\hat{\theta}_2 = 2.63$, and hence the patient should be allocated to outcome O_2. On the other hand, using the equations (6.10), the posterior probabilities of belonging to categories O_1, O_2, and O_3 are 46%, 21%, and 33%, respectively. Thus, the patient appears to have a greater chance to recover or to die than to remain severely disabled. The apparent contradiction between the predictions based on I and that derived from the posterior probabilities can be explained by the fact that whatever I-value, the posterior probability for outcome O_2 never exceeds 21%, i.e., the maximum value corresponding to $I = \frac{1}{2}(\hat{\theta}_1 + \hat{\theta}_2) = 2.21$. Thus, for each patient, the posterior probabilities for O_1 and O_3 will always exceed that for O_2. This problem has been discussed by Anderson and Philips (1981). It is recommended that prediction be based on the ratios of posterior to prior probabilities, which in the present case are $0.46/0.32 = 1.44$, $0.21/0.13 = 1.6$, and $0.33/0.55 = 0.6$, respectively, indicating that the patient is more likely to develop severe disability or a persistent vegetative state.

Applying the logistic model to the same patient population, but using CK-BB only, the risk index obtained was $I = 0.006212$ CK-BB and the thresholds were $\hat{\theta}_1 = 0.68$ (± 0.47) and $\hat{\theta}_2 = 1.44$ (± 0.50). Notice that $\hat{\theta}_1$ is not statistically different from zero, so that a two-outcome model (survival versus death) may be more appropriate in this case.

6.5 THE CONCEPT OF RESPONSE CURVES

In the preceding sections, methods were described for predicting outcomes from a single multivariate observation $\mathbf{x}$. In actual situations, however, serial measurements of the same variables are often available, and the question arises of how to use this accumulated information to assess the patient's risk. A typical problem in a coronary care unit consists of predicting the patient's chances of survival upon discharge from the hospital based on data collected repeatedly during hospitalization. The data may consist of daily determinations of serum creatine kinase (CK), blood urea, lactate dehydrogenase, etc. We can add to this information demographic characteristics recorded at admission, or other clinical information gained during the hospital stay. Thus, it is important to make a clear distinction between "baseline" variables measured only once (e.g., age, sex, weight, etc.) and "time-dependent" variables measured repeatedly (e.g., serial determination of biochemical constituents).

We consider the two-outcome prediction problem when the data consists of a mixture of baseline and time-dependent variables. The concept of a response curve is introduced, and a method is described for allocating a patient's response curve into one of two distinct groups or outcome categories.

Serial measurements of a single variable may be thought of as forming a response curve to the disease process, obtained simply by interpolating linearly between successive observations. For example, with acute myocardial infarction, there is typically a rise and fall of serum enzymes (see Figure 6.3). Both the shape and size of such response curves may bring valuable information for outcome prediction.

We will denote by

$$x(t) \qquad a \leq t \leq b \tag{6.12}$$

the response curve defined by the observation of variable X in the time period $[a,b]$. For example, $x(t)$ may represent the evolution of lactate dehydrogenase during the first ten days of acute care of a patient following myocardial infarction, or the evolution of C-reactive protein (CRP) during the first week after severe head injury.

Assume that instead of measuring one variable X, we observe repeatedly a profile of k tests $\mathbf{X}^T = (X_1, \ldots, X_k)$. Then the definition (6.12) extends immediately to

$$\mathbf{x}^T(t) = \{x_1(t), \ldots, x_k(t)\} \qquad a \leq t \leq b \tag{6.13}$$

which defines a "multivariate response curve" or "trajectory" in the $(k + 1)$-dimensional space, where each variable X_i corresponds to one coordinate axis and time t to another. For instance, in the acute myocardial infarction situation, $\mathbf{x}(t)$ may be the simultaneous observation of several biochemical

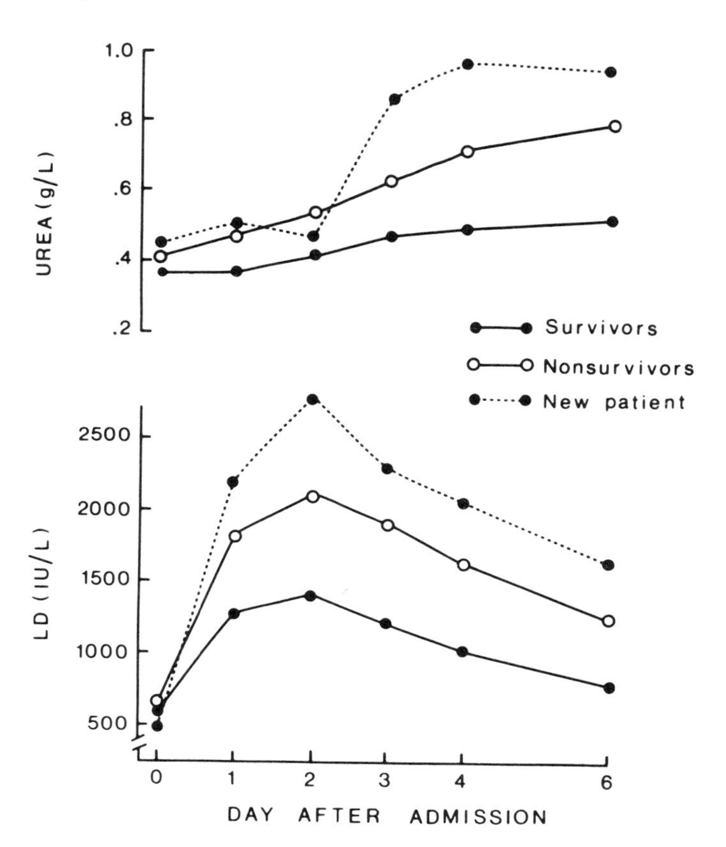

FIGURE 6.3 Average response curves of serum urea and lactate dehydrogenase (LD) in 120 survivors and 12 nonsurvivors (solid lines). The dotted line represents the response curve of a 70-year-old MI patient with no previous infarcts (see Table 6.3) (Albert, 1983).

constituents (LD, urea, CK, etc.) from admission ($a = 0$) until the end of hospitalization (e.g., $b = 15$ days).

The definition (6.13) is not restricted to time-dependent variables; constant parameters, such as age, can easily be made "time-dependent" by generating a dummy response curve, constant over the time interval considered. Thus $\mathbf{x}(t)$ defines a multivariate response curve, regardless of the nature

TABLE 6.3 Multivariate Series Recorded from a 70-Year-Old MI Patient with No Previous History of Myocardial Infarction (nMI = 0)

	Day after admission to the coronary-care unit					
Variables	0	1	2	3	4	6
Age (years)	70	70	70	70	70	70
nMI	0	0	0	0	0	0
Urea (g/L)	0.45	0.48	0.47	0.86	0.96	0.94
LD (U/L)	500	2238	2829	2319	2058	1620

of the variables considered, whether discrete or real-valued, time-dependent or not.

The example in Table 6.3 describes a one-week series of observations in a 70-year-old MI patient with no previous infarct. Linear interpolation between the six consecutive points produces a trajectory in five-dimensional space. The values of age and *nMI* are simply repeated at each time of observation. Of course, more sophisticated methods than simple linear interpolation may be used to derive the response curve, but this would require more complex theory and calculations that seem unjustified over a short time-span. Finally, there is no mathematical requirement that the serial measurements be recorded at equally spaced time points. As illustrated in the example above (Table 6.3), urea and LD were measured daily, except for day 5.

6.6 PROGNOSIS BASED ON RESPONSE CURVES

A. Distance Between Two Response Curves

Consider a sample of n patients suffering from disease D and suppose that for each patient the outcome, either O_1 or O_2, is known. Let n_1 and n_2 denote the numbers of patients with outcomes O_1 and O_2, respectively. Further, assume that the same variables have been measured in every patient at the same times during interval $[a,b]$. Denote by

$$\mathbf{x}_{ji}(t) \qquad a \leq t \leq b \qquad (j = 1,2;\ i = 1,n_j) \tag{6.14}$$

the observed response curve $\mathbf{x}^T(t) = \{x_1(t), \ldots, x_k(t)\}$ in the ith patient with outcome j.

We wish to construct an index for predicting a new patient's outcome when only his or her response curve is known. This situation is exactly similar to earlier prediction problems, except that here, outcome prediction is based on a response curve rather than a single multivariate observation. The concepts of discriminant analysis may be extended to the study of multivariate response curves (Albert, 1983). The basic idea is to classify a given patient's response curve to the group it resembles the most. Thus, for example, in acute myocardial infarction, it seems reasonable to consider a patient at high risk if his or her LD response curve during a hospital stay is closer to the average LD response curve of nonsurvivors than to that of survivors.

Closeness implies the notion of a distance between response curves. Consider two individuals and let $\mathbf{x}_1(t)$ and $\mathbf{x}_2(t)$ be their multivariate response curves in the time period $[a,b]$. We denote by $D(\mathbf{x}_1, \mathbf{x}_2)$ the distance between these curves. There are many ways to define distances and for algebraic reasons, it is often preferable to work with squared distances. The squared distance between $\mathbf{x}_1(t)$ and $\mathbf{x}_2(t)$ is defined by the relation

$$D^2(\mathbf{x}_1,\mathbf{x}_2) = (b - a)^{-1} \int_a^b \{\mathbf{x}_1(t) - \mathbf{x}_2(t)\}^T \mathbf{S}^{-1}(t) \{\mathbf{x}_1(t) - \mathbf{x}_2(t)\}\, dt \tag{6.15}$$

where $\mathbf{S}(t)$ is the covariance matrix of $\mathbf{X}$ at time t (sometimes called the metric). In (6.15) time disappears because the function is being integrated over the time span $[a,b]$. We note that distance is a single positive number, whereas response curves are multivariate time-dependent entities. So equation (6.15) takes us from the $(k + 1)$-dimensional space of response curves to the one-dimensional range of a univariate quantity.

B. Definition of Risk Index

Let $\bar{\mathbf{x}}_1(t)$ and $\bar{\mathbf{x}}_2(t)$ denote the average response curves for patients with outcomes O_1 and O_2, respectively. By definition,

$$\bar{\mathbf{x}}_j(t) = \frac{1}{n_j} \sum_{i=1}^{n_j} \mathbf{x}_{ji}(t) \tag{6.16}$$

Let $\mathbf{x}(t)$, $a \leq t \leq b$ denote the response curve of a patient with unknown outcome, and let $D^2(\mathbf{x},\bar{\mathbf{x}}_1)$ and $D^2(\mathbf{x},\bar{\mathbf{x}}_2)$ represent the distances between $\mathbf{x}(t)$ and the average response curves $\bar{\mathbf{x}}_1(t)$ and $\bar{\mathbf{x}}_2(t)$, as defined in (6.15).

To define the risk index, we proceed as follows. It is natural to allocate the patient to the outcome group O_1 if

$$D^2(\mathbf{x},\bar{\mathbf{x}}_1) \leq D^2(\mathbf{x},\bar{\mathbf{x}}_2) \tag{6.17}$$

that is, if the distance between $\mathbf{x}(t)$ and group O_1 is smaller than the distance between $\mathbf{x}(t)$ and group O_2.

The inequality (6.17) can also be written as

$$D^2(\mathbf{x},\bar{\mathbf{x}}_1) - D^2(\mathbf{x},\bar{\mathbf{x}}_2) \leq 0 \tag{6.18}$$

The left-hand side of (6.18), the difference between two positive numbers, can take any value, negative or positive, on the real line. Thus, it defines a risk index

$$I(\mathbf{x}) = D^2(\mathbf{x},\bar{\mathbf{x}}_1) - D^2(\mathbf{x},\bar{\mathbf{x}}_2) \tag{6.19}$$

because negative values of I are associated with outcome O_1 and positive values with outcome O_2. An index $I = 0$ would correspond to a multivariate response curve equally distant from the two outcome groups considered.

C. Efficiency of the Risk Index

Exactly as for classical discriminant analysis, one can calculate the index I for all patients of the training sample and record the number of patients predicted correctly. The percentage of correct predictions estimates the efficiency of the risk index.

Another way to proceed is to calculate the distance between the two average response curves $\overline{\mathbf{x}}_1(t)$ and $\overline{\mathbf{x}}_2(t), a \leq t \leq b$. The larger this distance $D^2(\overline{\mathbf{x}}_1, \overline{\mathbf{x}}_2)$, the better the dissociation between the two outcomes. At present, we have no way of assessing on a theoretical basis the significance of the group distance. There are no statistics for testing the hypothesis $D^2(\overline{\mathbf{x}}_1, \overline{\mathbf{x}}_2) = 0$, because the method described herein is purely descriptive. However, with only one time-dependent variable (univariate response curve), F-statistics proposed by Zerbe (1979) can be used to test the equality of mean response curves between the two groups. The Zerbe technique makes it possible to measure and assess the predictive ability of each time-dependent variable $x_1(t), \ldots, x_k(t)$ separately. The method does not apply when two or more variables are considered in a single multivariate response curve. Despite this restriction, the univariate approach often provides interesting information with respect to (1) selecting the best variables; and (2) discarding unnecessary or redundant variables.

D. Calculation of the Risk Index

The foregoing theory cannot generally be applied without making some assumptions and simplifications. We will assume that the variables $X_1, \ldots, X_k$ of the profile $\mathbf{X}$ are observed at q distinct time points, not necessarily equally distant, but the same for all patients. The response curve $\mathbf{x}(t)$ is obtained by linear interpolation. We may express this by writing $\mathbf{x}(t)$ in the form

$$\mathbf{x}(t) = \mathbf{Yc}(t) \qquad a \leq t \leq b \tag{6.20}$$

where $\mathbf{Y}$ is the $k \times q$ matrix of observations (e.g., Table 6.3), and $\mathbf{c}(t)$ is a time-dependent vector of length q defined in the intervals $[t_i,t_{i+1}]$, $(i = 1, \ldots, q - 1)$ by

$$\mathbf{c}^T(t) = (0, \ldots, 0, c_i, c_{i+1}, 0, \ldots, 0) \tag{6.21}$$

where

$$c_i = (t_{i+1} - t)/\Delta_i,\ c_{i+1} = (t - t_i)/\Delta_i \qquad \text{and}$$
$$\Delta_i = t_{i+1} - t_i$$

From the linear functional form (6.20) applied to all individual response curves, $\mathbf{x}_{ji}(t) = \mathbf{Y}_{ji}\mathbf{c}(t)$, $a \leq t \leq b$, $(j = 1,2;\ i = 1,n_j)$, Albert (1983) has shown that equation (6.19) becomes

$$I(\mathbf{x}) = (b - a)^{-1}\,\mathrm{tr}\,\{\mathbf{C}(\mathbf{A}^T\mathbf{Y} + \mathbf{B})\} \tag{6.22}$$

where "tr" is the trace matrix operator, i.e., the sum of the diagonal elements of the matrix, and

$$\begin{aligned} \mathbf{A}^T &= (\overline{\mathbf{Y}}_2 - \overline{\mathbf{Y}}_1)^T\mathbf{S}^{-1} \\ \mathbf{B} &= -{}^1\!/_2\mathbf{A}^T(\overline{\mathbf{Y}}_1 + \overline{\mathbf{Y}}_2) \end{aligned} \tag{6.23}$$

In the above expressions, $\overline{\mathbf{Y}}_1$ and $\overline{\mathbf{Y}}_2$ are the matrices of mean values of all variables at all times in groups O_1 and O_2, respectively,

$$\mathbf{S} = \frac{\sum_{j=1}^{2}\sum_{i=1}^{n_j}(\mathbf{Y}_{ji} - \overline{\mathbf{Y}}_j)\,\mathbf{C}\,(\mathbf{Y}_{ji} - \overline{\mathbf{Y}}_j)^T}{\{(n_1 + n_2 - 2)(b - a)\}} \tag{6.24}$$

and $\mathbf{C}$ is a q-dimensional symmetric matrix with all elements equal to zero except those directly below and above the diagonal line which are given by

$$C_{ii} = \frac{\Delta_{i-1} + \Delta_i}{3}$$
$$C_{i,i+1} = C_{i+1,i} = \frac{\Delta_i}{6} \tag{6.25}$$

In summary, although the formulas above are somewhat complex, the procedure is fairly simple, as follows:

1. Determine $\overline{\mathbf{Y}}_1$ and $\overline{\mathbf{Y}}_2$, the matrices of the mean values of all variables at all times in groups O_1 and O_2, respectively.
2. Determine matrix $\mathbf{C}$.
3. Calculate the covariance matrix $\mathbf{S}$.
4. Determine the coefficient matrices $\mathbf{A}$ and $\mathbf{B}$, using equations (6.23).
5. Calculate the risk index I for the new patient using formula (6.22), which involves only matrix manipulations and summations.

6.7 APPLICATION TO PROGNOSIS AFTER ACUTE MYOCARDIAL INFARCTION

To illustrate these procedures, this analysis of multivariate response curves was applied to data from a study of 132 patients with acute myocardial infarction (Albert, 1983). There were 120 still alive a month after MI (group O_1) and 12 who had died within a month (group O_2). For each patient, age and number of previous infarctions (*nMI*) were recorded at admission ($t = 0$). Two serum constituents, lactate dehydrogenase (LD, U/L) and serum urea (g/L), were measured daily during the first four days and on day 6 ($t = 6$). All data are listed in

TABLE 6.4 Means ± SD of Urea and LD Levels in Survivors ($n = 120$) and Nonsurvivors ($n = 12$) at Each Time Point

Time (days)	Urea (g/L)		LD (U/L)	
	Survivors	Non-survivors	Survivors	Non-survivors
0	0.37 ± 0.09	0.42 ± 0.22	566 ± 259	576 ± 337
1	0.37 ± 0.12	0.48 ± 0.27	1329 ± 571	1843 ± 444
2	0.41 ± 0.13	0.54 ± 0.31	1433 ± 628	2149 ± 555
3	0.47 ± 0.14	0.63 ± 0.36	1272 ± 565	1901 ± 631
4	0.49 ± 0.15	0.72 ± 0.40	1046 ± 425	1636 ± 469
6	0.51 ± 0.15	0.79 ± 0.39	821 ± 311	1280 ± 330
F-test[a]	14.90		14.94	
Degrees of freedom	($\nu_1 = 1.1$, $\nu_2 = 140.7$)		($\nu_1 = 1.2$, $\nu_2 = 158.3$)	
Significance	$p < 0.001$		$p < 0.001$	

[a]F-values of the comparison of the average response curves between the two groups over the one-week investigation period. In contrast to classical statistical F-tests, the degrees of freedom for Zerbe's F-test are fractional and calculated from the data themselves and the length of the investigation period.

Source: Albert (1983).

Appendix II. The variables age (survivors: 55.5 ± 8.8 years; nonsurvivors: 62.2 ± 8.8 years, $p < 0.01$) and *nMI* (survivors: 0.26 ± 0.64; nonsurvivors: 0.67 ± 0.78, $p < 0.05$) are known to be important for short-term prognosis. The average response curves of LD and urea (Table 6.4 and Figure 6.3) in survivors and nonsurvivors were compared separately using Zerbe's method. Both F-values were highly significant, emphasizing the importance of these two constituents in defining a risk index for myocardial infarction.

Proceeding on this basis, the matrix $\mathbf{Y}$ [equation (6.20)] for each patient has four rows (age, *nMI*, urea, and LD) and six columns (days after admission). Thus, $k = 4$, $q = 6$, $a = 0$ and $b = 6$. The matrix $\mathbf{C}$ and the covariance matrix $\mathbf{S}$,

TABLE 6.5 Linear Interpolation Coefficient Matrix **C**, Calculated from Equations (6.25)[a]

Time points	Time points 0	1	2	3	4	6
0	0.3333					
1	0.1667	0.6667				
2		0.1667	0.6667			
3			0.1667	0.6667		
4				0.1667	1.0	
6					0.3333	0.6667

[a]All nonprinted elements of the matrix are zeroes.

TABLE 6.6 Weighted Covariance Matrix **S** [Equation (6.24)] over the Six-Day Period for the Four Variables Studied[a]

	Age	nMI	Urea	LD
Age	76.9			
nMI	0.217	0.428		
Urea	0.345	−0.0063	0.0253	
LD	−435	−33.8	5.25	225043

[a]Age, number of previous infarctions, serum urea, and lactate dehydrogenase.

weighted over the six-day period, are given in Tables 6.5 and 6.6.

Table 6.7 displays the elements of the weight matrix **A** [equation (6.23)] computed from the data. The elements of **B** [equation (6.23)] obtained from those of **A**, are given in Table 6.8. Owing to the special form of the matrix **C**, only the diagonal elements of **B** and those directly above and below the diagonal line are needed. Table 6.7 shows that all weights are positive, indicating that high parameter values are a sign of poor prognosis. The matrix of correlations among the four tests, pooled over the one-week period, did not reveal large correlations, except perhaps for *nMI* and urea ($r = 0.25$).

TABLE 6.7 Coefficient Matrix **A** [Equation (6.23)] Derived from a Sample of 132 MI Patients (120 Survivors, 12 Nonsurvivors)

Time points (days)	Variables			
	Age	nMI	Urea	LD ($\times 10^{-4}$)
0	0.08	0.95	1.03	3
1	0.08	1.15	2.91	26
2	0.09	1.23	3.38	35
3	0.08	1.22	4.83	30
4	0.06	1.25	7.95	27
6	0.05	1.24	10.15	21

Source: Albert (1983).

TABLE 6.8 Matrix **B** of Intercept Elements [Equation (6.23)] Derived from a Sample of 132 MI Patients (120 Survivors, 12 Nonsurvivors)

Time points (days)	Time points (days)					
	0	1	2	3	4	6
0	−5.80	−6.16				
1	−8.11	−10.82	−11.47			
2		−12.65	−13.50	−13.05		
3			−12.87	−12.62	−12.14	
4				−12.98	−12.74	−12.33
6					−12.38	−12.26

A risk index was calculated for each patient and the number of correct and incorrect predictions recorded. Results are displayed in Table 6.9. The cut point chosen for allocating patients to one or the other group was $I = 0$.

It follows that the global specificity (correctly predicted survivors) and sensitivity (correctly predicted nonsurvivors) are 85% (102/120) and 83.3% (10/12), respectively. Assuming a death rate of 15%, the predictive value of a positive index is 50%. In other words, a positive index multiplies the risk of

TABLE 6.9 Prediction Matrix Derived from a Sample of 132 MI Patients

	True outcome	
	Survivors (n = 120)	Nonsurvivors (n = 12)
Predicted outcome		
Low risk[a]: $I \leq 0$	102	2
High risk[a]: $I > 0$	18	10

[a]The risk index I is based on age, number of previous infarctions, urea, and LD serial concentrations over a six-day period.

death by a factor of 3. On the other hand, the predictive value of a negative index is 94%, almost ruling out the possibility of death.

Finally, the calculation of the risk index for the patient given in Table 6.3 yields a score of 2.88, indicating unfavorable prognosis. As seen from Figure 6.3, from day 2 after admission, urea and LD concentrations are well above average levels recorded in nonsurvivors. Actually, the patient died 11 days after admission to the coronary care unit.

6.8 FINAL REMARKS

The statistical methods described in this chapter, whether logistic, probit, or based on multivariate response curves, have been designed to derive risk indices and predict outcomes of a particular disease from a set of clinical and laboratory data. They require few distributional assumptions about the variables involved, discrete, continuous, or a mixture of both, and therefore apply to many prognostic problems arising in daily practice. In addition to robustness, the methods exhibit simplicity and feasibility. The indices are simple linear combinations of the risk factors, and the posterior probabilities easily obtained even on pocket or desk-top calculators. Finally, the variable selection procedures described for medical diagnosis (Chapter 5) can be extended to prognosis. Thus, variables bringing repetitious information can be discarded and those immediately related to outcome and providing jointly the best predictive efficiency can be selected on a statistically sound basis.

Despite many interesting features, prognostic indices have a major shortcoming, they provide only a "pointwise" assessment of the patient's condition and do not emphasize the dynamics of the disease process. The coefficients of the risk index are calculated only once, after a fixed monitoring period. Some patients may die before the end of this fixed interval and thus be omitted from the database. Likewise, a patient's status may suddenly improve or deteriorate and his or her chances of survival change dramatically at any time during the fixed period before the index would be computed. The response curve method developed in Sections 6.5 and 6.6 suffers from the same defect. Serial data are not used in a dynamic way but viewed as a fixed entity, and complete knowledge of the response curve is necessary to make a prognosis. A dynamic statistical treatment and adequate interpretation of serial laboratory determinations will be discussed in the next chapter.

APPENDIX I: SEVERE HEAD INJURY DATA

OUTCOME 1 Favorable Evolution
(Good Recovery or Moderate Disability)

Patient	Outcome	Age	CK-BB
1	1	19	100
2	1	11	220
3	1	38	6
4	1	7	281
5	1	17	17
6	1	19	27
7	1	12	96

OUTCOME 1 Favorable Evolution (cont'd.)
(Good Recovery or Moderate Disability)

Patient	Outcome	Age	CK-BB
8	1	8	23
9	1	24	253
10	1	16	60
11	1	18	126
12	1	12	100
13	1	8	200
14	1	28	70
15	1	10	146
16	1	46	46
17	1	35	40
18	1	6	136
19	1	6	286

OUTCOME 2 Unfavorable Evolution
(Severe Disability or Persistent Vegetative State)

Patient	Outcome	Age	CK-BB
20	2	8	230
21	2	23	509
22	2	19	283
23	2	4	140
24	2	29	80
25	2	23	576
26	2	20	76
27	2	62	206

OUTCOME 3 Death

Patient	Outcome	Age	CK-BB
28	3	17	253
29	3	29	490
30	3	7	1087
31	3	59	76
32	3	61	303

OUTCOME 3 Death (cont'd.)

Patient	Outcome	Age	CK-BB
33	3	45	1560
34	3	61	353
35	3	20	1370
36	3	24	671
37	3	22	60
38	3	30	356
39	3	20	543
40	3	45	120
41	3	16	700
42	3	16	16
43	3	50	216
44	3	16	800
45	3	19	90
46	3	19	303
47	3	11	183
48	3	18	740
49	3	15	1256
50	3	56	523
51	3	40	350
52	3	18	126
53	3	18	153
54	3	20	913
55	3	19	193
56	3	41	323
57	3	51	443
58	3	29	156
59	3	21	463
60	3	20	230

Source: Reproduced by permission of P. Hans, M.D., and J.D. Born, M.D.

APPENDIX II: ACUTE MYOCARDIAL INFARCTION DATA

OUTCOME 1 Survival

				Urea (g/L)						LD (U/L)					
				Day after admission						Day after admission					
Pt.	Out-come	Age	nMI	0	1	2	3	4	6	0	1	2	3	4	6
1	1	59	2	0.55	0.55	0.40	0.44	0.49	0.58	708	1016	1479	1240	766	526
2	1	56	0	0.31	0.31	0.38	0.32	0.40	0.54	683	966	760	790	700	413
3	1	50	0	0.58	0.52	0.50	0.52	0.51	0.72	400	1310	1370	1253	1040	825
4	1	68	0	0.48	0.48	0.40	0.44	0.48	0.52	400	1003	1270	1253	1016	780
5	1	59	0	0.32	0.26	0.22	0.28	0.33	0.38	400	1106	1436	1160	1010	860
6	1	57	0	0.32	0.32	0.40	0.40	0.45	0.46	400	1260	700	673	580	500
7	1	55	0	0.42	0.38	0.34	0.45	0.55	0.66	400	1110	1283	1150	1000	650
8	1	66	2	0.40	0.32	0.38	0.44	0.41	0.42	400	1671	1247	523	527	343
9	1	68	1	0.44	0.54	0.50	0.66	0.62	0.80	400	3335	2949	2181	1941	1367
10	1	48	0	0.25	0.20	0.20	0.34	0.42	0.61	400	1000	1143	1290	873	687
11	1	65	1	0.30	0.28	0.62	0.49	0.50	0.36	954	1509	1463	1329	1126	833
12	1	48	0	0.47	0.57	0.68	0.62	0.58	0.58	1004	1608	1396	1110	1030	563
13	1	63	0	0.40	0.34	0.74	0.77	0.79	0.62	1200	2108	1968	1440	1136	743
14	1	57	0	0.42	0.45	0.54	0.59	0.60	0.64	400	653	636	590	506	448
15	1	69	0	0.37	0.32	0.39	0.43	0.46	0.46	910	1420	1386	1263	1350	1032
16	1	51	0	0.38	0.42	0.42	0.62	0.56	0.49	400	546	564	583	521	460
17	1	60	0	0.20	0.24	0.26	0.32	0.34	0.32	350	553	590	390	350	300
18	1	75	0	0.40	0.52	0.46	0.32	0.38	0.37	400	853	1046	1033	963	913
19	1	44	0	0.40	0.30	0.30	0.47	0.64	0.65	450	2458	2400	2199	1909	1620
20	1	60	1	0.48	0.45	0.57	0.58	0.60	0.60	733	810	633	423	390	350
21	1	57	0	0.54	0.61	0.63	0.71	0.64	0.60	450	1788	2760	2538	2010	1440
22	1	56	0	0.50	0.54	0.33	0.49	0.42	0.45	400	1136	1373	1140	1070	800
23	1	50	0	0.50	0.61	0.72	0.70	0.64	0.61	583	920	823	800	603	596
24	1	48	0	0.32	0.54	0.52	0.46	0.50	0.50	923	1423	1223	963	886	736
25	1	55	0	0.26	0.20	0.40	0.60	0.49	0.50	500	1086	1310	1809	1183	776
26	1	59	0	0.28	0.29	0.31	0.31	0.31	0.38	350	498	422	346	276	343
27	1	50	0	0.35	0.37	0.31	0.43	0.56	0.46	400	1045	1509	1488	1266	776
28	1	43	0	0.26	0.26	0.27	0.30	0.28	0.34	914	1428	1060	853	776	566
29	1	53	4	0.32	0.26	0.32	0.32	0.36	0.40	400	966	1036	670	710	570
30	1	51	0	0.30	0.30	0.38	0.37	0.29	0.39	416	443	530	430	436	499
31	1	66	0	0.44	0.40	0.48	0.51	0.63	0.77	450	1166	1968	1968	1968	1216
32	1	45	0	0.48	0.52	0.60	0.77	0.79	1.26	650	2700	3365	2760	2079	1548
33	1	51	0	0.40	0.40	0.40	0.42	0.50	0.50	350	476	436	590	538	485
34	1	68	0	0.28	0.29	0.30	0.36	0.30	0.30	906	1401	1256	1098	940	750
35	1	51	0	0.34	0.29	0.36	0.47	0.54	0.76	400	2298	2250	1869	1380	973
36	1	46	0	0.35	0.41	0.48	0.55	0.50	0.47	1578	1908	1740	1303	1066	834
37	1	78	0	0.36	0.40	0.56	0.50	0.64	0.60	350	610	673	716	663	610
38	1	48	1	0.44	0.40	0.36	0.36	0.57	0.60	1220	2040	1407	1220	800	650
39	1	61	0	0.38	0.44	0.54	0.54	0.66	0.60	905	1410	1470	1320	1048	776

OUTCOME 1 Survival (*continued*)

				Urea (g/L)						LD (U/L)					
				Day after admission						Day after admission					
Pt.	Out-come	Age	nMI	0	1	2	3	4	6	0	1	2	3	4	6
40	1	56	0	0.32	0.18	0.20	0.26	0.40	0.28	400	1971	2109	1578	1300	1016
41	1	56	3	0.30	0.28	0.46	0.60	0.64	0.46	400	983	1100	1016	813	593
42	1	65	0	0.49	0.84	0.90	0.86	0.77	0.69	400	691	750	820	623	540
43	1	32	0	0.30	0.25	0.24	0.30	0.30	0.30	400	2460	2259	2388	1638	1250
44	1	66	0	0.45	0.45	0.37	0.62	0.64	0.63	1025	1650	1650	1581	1350	1123
45	1	33	0	0.24	0.24	0.30	0.46	0.50	0.49	486	573	570	436	396	338
46	1	66	1	0.36	0.38	0.62	0.74	0.88	0.54	1059	1719	1938	1770	1280	900
47	1	67	1	0.31	0.50	0.66	0.76	0.88	1.10	520	590	700	560	555	553
48	1	46	0	0.26	0.17	0.27	0.36	0.40	0.52	400	1036	990	1063	920	636
49	1	43	0	0.33	0.44	0.36	0.47	0.44	0.41	450	1860	2049	1710	1363	1010
50	1	62	0	0.28	0.28	0.19	0.48	0.36	0.46	350	616	900	1260	1210	933
51	1	54	0	0.30	0.33	0.32	0.40	0.39	0.38	450	1147	1277	1220	950	800
52	1	59	0	0.30	0.48	0.49	0.51	0.50	0.48	493	670	783	600	660	600
53	1	47	0	0.30	0.19	0.24	0.42	0.41	0.40	450	2259	2388	2208	1549	1182
54	1	63	0	0.30	0.40	0.51	0.62	0.86	0.80	600	2280	2358	2049	2103	1602
55	1	53	0	0.40	0.50	0.55	0.60	0.66	0.74	730	746	676	606	528	450
56	1	55	0	0.48	0.30	0.39	0.51	0.46	0.45	550	2019	2418	2250	1740	1360
57	1	57	0	0.28	0.30	0.43	0.42	0.42	0.42	400	613	750	627	513	480
58	1	53	0	0.38	0.43	0.48	0.79	0.88	0.85	400	1250	1680	1509	1146	964
59	1	39	0	0.18	0.28	0.38	0.36	0.39	0.38	776	756	736	496	436	436
60	1	68	0	0.19	0.38	0.28	0.38	0.48	0.44	450	1346	1710	1286	926	750
61	1	54	0	0.46	0.46	0.43	0.44	0.47	0.50	400	1053	860	760	633	546
62	1	34	1	0.32	0.28	0.32	0.49	0.54	0.50	400	986	936	730	576	423
63	1	59	0	0.29	0.30	0.48	0.69	0.68	0.67	1044	2850	3078	2928	1818	1414
64	1	56	0	0.36	0.47	0.77	0.70	0.56	0.61	930	2238	2118	1818	1443	1650
65	1	69	0	0.27	0.46	0.45	0.42	0.44	0.46	400	1488	2019	1809	1504	1200
66	1	54	0	0.54	0.40	0.46	0.53	0.70	0.76	400	1196	1183	876	794	712
67	1	72	0	0.38	0.38	0.62	0.75	0.82	0.82	836	946	916	856	886	724
68	1	58	0	0.36	0.26	0.43	0.43	0.42	0.52	400	1740	1433	1240	950	943
69	1	42	0	0.30	0.42	0.48	0.51	0.54	0.56	450	1659	1878	1909	1454	1000
70	1	54	0	0.28	0.36	0.54	0.52	0.49	0.44	450	2118	2199	2190	1400	1050
71	1	66	0	0.26	0.36	0.31	0.36	0.32	0.32	678	1103	1090	836	793	662
72	1	54	0	0.50	0.45	0.40	0.42	0.44	0.52	676	1264	1456	1196	1056	916
73	1	60	0	0.52	0.46	0.40	0.37	0.38	0.38	1119	1839	1749	1520	1306	1004
74	1	45	0	0.32	0.24	0.20	0.24	0.33	0.42	906	1406	1203	1263	1083	756
75	1	61	0	0.28	0.51	0.40	0.44	0.44	0.48	400	1533	2088	1878	1488	1100
76	1	53	1	0.30	0.31	0.40	0.47	0.46	0.46	651	903	946	853	680	560
77	1	58	0	0.36	0.24	0.33	0.52	0.46	0.42	400	1728	1950	1599	1213	823
78	1	47	0	0.36	0.27	0.26	0.35	0.32	0.32	1014	1920	2280	1608	1360	1040
79	1	57	0	0.40	0.30	0.32	0.38	0.32	0.42	400	656	976	1006	740	556
80	1	50	0	0.25	0.19	0.25	0.42	0.45	0.42	1030	1280	1336	1336	966	796
81	1	52	0	0.33	0.35	0.43	0.52	0.45	0.52	551	1650	1950	1668	1296	1013

Outcome 1 Survival (*continued*)

Pt.	Out-come	Age	nMI	Urea (g/L) Day after admission 0	1	2	3	4	6	LD (U/L) Day after admission 0	1	2	3	4	6
82	1	47	2	0.30	0.38	0.26	0.28	0.30	0.47	400	946	1276	1376	1433	988
83	1	49	0	0.44	0.41	0.53	0.66	0.66	0.50	400	1629	2550	2778	1998	1233
84	1	49	0	0.44	0.36	0.61	0.72	0.71	0.72	450	1769	2130	2019	1749	1353
85	1	48	0	0.36	0.32	0.32	0.35	0.36	0.49	400	1233	1590	1476	1313	1206
86	1	51	0	0.52	0.48	0.44	0.37	0.36	0.36	400	1788	1758	1433	1176	920
87	1	62	0	0.40	0.58	0.44	0.52	0.48	0.58	400	876	1083	993	843	750
88	1	50	0	0.27	0.32	0.34	0.47	0.38	0.34	500	630	656	663	516	440
89	1	49	0	0.32	0.34	0.46	0.51	0.45	0.45	400	1157	1929	1950	1563	1230
90	1	69	0	0.34	0.37	0.43	0.35	0.45	0.49	450	1346	1638	1486	1383	1093
91	1	53	0	0.25	0.24	0.52	0.52	0.45	0.51	630	1260	1240	830	943	500
92	1	60	0	0.48	0.42	0.42	0.48	0.49	0.48	480	580	570	520	450	400
92	1	52	0	0.52	0.42	0.32	0.44	0.49	0.43	400	1280	1509	1483	1173	863
94	1	66	1	0.36	0.40	0.40	0.52	0.57	0.55	400	1070	1220	1363	1070	800
95	1	70	1	0.48	0.44	0.46	0.66	0.78	0.75	686	1106	1130	1150	883	683
96	1	57	0	0.50	0.34	0.40	0.42	0.44	0.51	400	906	783	676	670	540
97	1	66	0	0.30	0.32	0.28	0.28	0.28	0.36	986	1166	1090	928	837	863
98	1	53	0	0.38	0.26	0.31	0.38	0.45	0.47	450	797	1053	773	663	586
99	1	64	1	0.38	0.50	0.34	0.32	0.34	0.37	357	817	777	580	550	496
100	1	56	0	0.26	0.44	0.32	0.28	0.40	0.46	300	1223	1698	1770	1890	1195
101	1	57	0	0.22	0.24	0.26	0.27	0.29	0.31	350	843	896	803	786	593
102	1	50	0	0.34	0.30	0.36	0.33	0.30	0.32	400	796	1016	753	780	783
103	1	60	0	0.42	0.46	0.44	0.56	0.66	0.68	848	1659	1869	1659	1123	1120
104	1	58	1	0.30	0.22	0.24	0.32	0.32	0.38	820	1980	1638	1569	1286	913
105	1	54	0	0.35	0.37	0.40	0.45	0.50	0.50	350	866	733	676	540	420
106	1	68	1	0.24	0.40	0.48	0.40	0.40	0.40	800	1483	1067	963	790	783
107	1	51	1	0.40	0.48	0.42	0.50	0.40	0.40	730	1869	1920	1518	1130	913
108	1	64	0	0.24	0.24	0.30	0.34	0.34	0.42	727	1077	1036	840	746	516
109	1	49	1	0.42	0.26	0.22	0.40	0.38	0.38	400	993	1106	933	836	516
110	1	58	1	0.48	0.32	0.23	0.28	0.29	0.39	450	997	1103	1017	907	797
111	1	45	0	0.38	0.38	0.36	0.38	0.38	0.40	250	1210	1680	1511	1343	1153
112	1	55	0	0.55	0.42	0.40	0.44	0.48	0.46	450	2040	2280	1638	1310	1183
113	1	43	0	0.27	0.29	0.30	0.32	0.32	0.44	300	717	637	643	463	470
114	1	59	0	0.43	0.40	0.38	0.42	0.46	0.51	300	1941	2049	1770	1167	900
115	1	49	0	0.32	0.24	0.28	0.40	0.38	0.43	1143	2679	2640	1920	1437	1033
116	1	51	0	0.48	0.38	0.42	0.51	0.53	0.57	350	997	1370	1260	1035	810
117	1	53	0	0.30	0.26	0.28	0.28	0.34	0.41	1073	1350	1380	1153	1079	1006
118	1	36	0	0.25	0.26	0.27	0.32	0.32	0.38	300	1403	2265	2010	1511	1013
119	1	52	2	0.44	0.42	0.36	0.29	0.36	0.57	350	1120	1320	1303	927	617
120	1	68	0	0.50	0.75	0.77	0.78	0.63	0.57	400	2001	2500	1779	1346	1296

Outcome 2 Death

Pt.	Out-come	Age	NMI	Urea (g/L) Day after admission 0	1	2	3	4	6	LD (U/L) Day after admission 0	1	2	3	4	6
121	2	48	2	0.39	0.45	0.50	0.58	0.60	0.63	1275	2151	2640	2190	1852	1177
122	2	65	2	0.34	0.32	0.30	0.32	0.32	0.46	400	1443	1911	1791	1530	920
123	2	64	0	0.54	0.48	0.41	0.49	0.56	0.74	818	1835	1989	1206	1183	1126
124	2	50	0	0.38	0.42	0.58	0.76	0.64	0.60	1164	2349	2640	2250	2058	1629
125	2	64	1	1.04	1.24	1.17	0.95	1.01	0.68	650	843	1116	746	700	533
126	2	60	0	0.45	0.48	0.47	0.86	0.96	0.94	500	2238	2829	2319	2058	1620
127	2	62	0	0.25	0.25	0.25	0.27	0.34	0.79	350	1728	1950	1569	1404	1238
128	2	64	1	0.34	0.32	0.30	0.36	0.49	0.56	350	2031	2361	2631	2169	1689
129	2	53	1	0.26	0.34	0.56	0.52	0.52	0.52	350	2279	2838	2739	2190	1533
130	2	70	0	0.35	0.27	0.22	0.26	0.50	0.69	300	2130	1809	1680	1578	1333
131	2	66	1	0.22	0.58	0.56	0.61	0.89	0.90	350	1569	2319	2469	1779	1326
132	2	80	0	0.42	0.64	1.10	1.52	1.76	1.94	400	1518	1383	1223	1130	1240

Source: Reproduced by permission of J. P. Chapelle, Ph.D.

REFERENCES

Albert, A. (1983). Discriminant analysis based on multivariate response curves: a descriptive approach to dynamic allocation. *Stat. Med. 2*, 95–106.

Albert, A., and Anderson, J. A. (1981). Probit and logistic discriminant functions. *Commun. Statist. A10*, 641–657.

Albert, A., Chapelle, J. P., and Smeets, J. P. (1981). Stepwise probit discrimination with specific application to short-term prognosis in acute myocardial infarction. *Comp. Biom. Res. 14*, 371–378.

Anderson, J. A., and Philips, P. R. (1981). Regression, discrimination and measurement models for ordered categorical data. *Appl. Statist. 30*, 22–31.

Chapelle, J. P., Albert, A., Kulbertus, H. E., and Heusghem, C. (1983). The long-term prognostic significance of biochemical measurements obtained during the acute phase of myocardial infarction. In *The First Year After a Myocardial Infarction*, H. E. Kulbertus and H. J. J. Willems (Eds.). Futura Publishing Company, Mount Kisco, New York, pp. 15–26.

Chapelle, J. P., Albert, A., Smeets, J. P., Demoulin, J. C., Foidart, G., Boland, J., Heusghem, C., and Kulbertus, H. E. (1981). Early assessment of risk in patients with acute myocardial infarction. *Eur. Heart J. 2*, 187–196.

Finney, D. J. (1971). *Probit Analysis*. 3rd edition. Cambridge University Press, Cambridge.
Hans, P., Albert, A., Born, J. D., and Chapelle, J. P. (1985). Derivation of a bioclinical index in severe head injury. *Int. Care Med. 11*, 186–191.
Jennett, B., and Bond, M. (1975). Assessment of outcome after severe brain damage. *Lancet 1*, 480–484.
Zerbe, G. O. (1979). Randomization analysis of the completely randomized design extended to growth and response curves. *J. Am. Stat. Assoc. 74*, 215–221.

7

THE DYNAMIC APPROACH TO PROGNOSIS

7.1
INTRODUCTION

Serial measurements are now a natural part of laboratory medicine. Thus, when a patient under severe stress is admitted to an intensive care unit, such as after a heart attack, burn, or shock trauma, he or she is submitted to a panel of clinical laboratory tests that are systematically repeated throughout hospitalization. This yields a huge amount of information that needs to be integrated and interpreted by the physician for monitoring and decision-making purposes. Among the various laboratory tests performed, some are likely to present repetitious information. As to those chemistries that truly reflect the patient's status, it is questionable whether the serial measurements recorded are used optimally for outcome prediction. Continuous risk assessment and day-to-day outcome prediction from the cumulative laboratory data collected during the patient's stay remain a challenging statistical problem.

So far, we have looked at medical prognosis from a "static" point of view. Patients were classified into two outcome categories (survival and death), and prediction was based on a single multivariate observation or response curve. No account was made for actual survival time, since nonsurvivors were grouped regardless of whether they had died soon after admission to the hospital or much later.

This chapter goes a step further by regarding prognosis as a dynamic process and describing three statistical methods that account for the temporal changes in the pathophysiological process of the disease. The first, a "brute force" technique, calculates a risk index at each time point, using, for example, the logistic model described in Section 6.2. The second is a straightforward extension of the response curve method developed in Section 6.6. The third method is conceptually more satisfactory and probably more useful. It extends the theory of risk indices to time-dependent outcome and covariates, leading to the concept of a "dynamic" risk index. It applies to any disease in which there is an acute phase during which the patient is closely monitored and multiple serial measurements are made. In acute diseases, as opposed to stable disease processes (Chapter 8), biochemical constituents do not always fluctuate around some threshold value but often follow a typical deterministic pattern (e.g., characteristic rise and fall of serum enzymes after MI). Elimination of this deterministic component from the observed time series is necessary to achieve stationarity, that is, to obtain a dynamic risk index with constant coefficients.

7.2 NOTATION AND PROBLEM FORMULATION

Consider a vector of laboratory tests $\mathbf{X}^T = (X_1, \ldots, X_k)$ and denote by $\mathbf{x}(t)$ the observed value at time t, $\mathbf{x}(t - 1)$ at time $t - 1$, and so on back to some starting point $t = 0$ (e.g., admission).

Let Y_t be the outcome variable in the time interval $[t, t + 1]$. For example, in the two-outcome case of survival versus nonsurvival, $y_t = 1$ if the patient is still alive at time $t + 1$, and $y_t = 2$ if he or she dies in this interval.

We define the "past" of the patient at time t as the grand vector $\mathbf{U}(t)$ of all information available for the patient at time t, namely, the observed profiles $\mathbf{x}(t)$, $\mathbf{x}(t - 1)$, and so on. Thus,

$$\begin{aligned} \mathbf{U}_t^T &= \{\mathbf{x}^T(t), \mathbf{x}^T(t - 1), \ldots\} \qquad \text{and} \\ \mathbf{U}_{t+1}^T &= \{\mathbf{x}^T(t + 1), \mathbf{U}_t^T\} \end{aligned} \tag{7.1}$$

The above definitions require some comment. First, they assume that observations are made at regular time intervals, e.g., every hour, day, or week. This is not necessarily true, in which case the time points will be explicitly noted $t_1, t_2, \ldots,$ etc. Second, the notation $\mathbf{x}(t)$, $a \leq t \leq b$, still defines a continuous multivariate response curve between the time points a and b, as in Section 6.5. Finally, if baseline variables are considered, they are measured only once and we assume that their values are added to the observation vector $\mathbf{x}(0)$ recorded at $t = 0$.

The statistical problem consists of predicting outcome Y_t from the patient's past vector $\mathbf{U}_t$. We should like to derive a linear, time-related ("dynamic") risk index $I(t)$

$$I(t) = a_0(t) + \mathbf{a}_1^T(t)\mathbf{x}(t) + \mathbf{a}_2^T(t)\mathbf{x}(t-1) + \cdots \qquad (7.2)$$

from which we may assess the patient's outcome probabilities $\text{pr}(y_t = 1|\mathbf{U}_t)$ and $\text{pr}(y_t = 2|\mathbf{U}_t)$, for $t = 0, 1, 2, \ldots$ in a two-outcome problem. The coefficients $\mathbf{a}_1$, $\mathbf{a}_2$, etc., are themselves time-dependent vectors of dimension k, since $\mathbf{x}(t)$, $\mathbf{x}(t-1)$, $\ldots$, are vectors. Thus, the equation of the risk index $I(t)$ is generally different at each time point.

Associated with the development of a dynamic prognostic index $I(t)$, there is a two-fold data selection problem:

1. Which variable(s), baseline or time-dependent, should enter the index?
2. How much past information is required at each time t?

For example, it may be that only part of the laboratory profile should be measured regularly, because of the repetitiousness of some of the tests. This question is similar to the variable selection problem discussed in previous chapters. The second question, however, is new and specific to time-dependent information. In some circumstances, it may be that only the most recent observation $\mathbf{x}(t)$ is sufficient for assessing the patient's condition, or that the last two observations $\mathbf{x}(t)$ and $\mathbf{x}(t-1)$ are needed; in another situation, the whole past may be required. Experience shows that quite often the former case holds, leading to a simplified form of equation (7.2).

7.3 THE REPEATED LOGISTIC METHOD

The crudest method for solving the dynamic outcome prediction problem is to perform a classical discriminant analysis at each time point, using, for example, the logistic model as in Section 6.2.

Assume that at time t, there are $n(t)$ patients and let $\mathbf{x}_i(t)$ denote the value of the profile observed for the ith patient ($i = 1, \ldots, n_t$). It is known that after time t, $n_1(t)$ patients will eventually have outcome O_1 while $n_2(t)$ will have outcome O_2.

By applying logistic discrimination to the sample data, one obtains a linear risk index

$$\begin{aligned} I(t) &= a_0(t) + a_1(t)x_1(t) + \cdots + a_k(t)x_k(t) \\ &= a_0(t) + \mathbf{a}^T(t)\mathbf{x}(t) \end{aligned} \tag{7.3}$$

which may then be calculated for every new patient for whom data are available at time t. The corresponding probability of developing the less favorable outcome O_2 is given by the logistic relation

$$\text{pr}\{O_2|\mathbf{x}(t)\} = \frac{\exp\{I(t)\}}{1 + \exp\{I(t)\}} \tag{7.4}$$

and

$$\text{pr}\{O_1|\mathbf{x}(t)\} = 1 - \text{pr}\{O_2|\mathbf{x}(t)\}$$

At some later point in time $t' > t$, the procedure can be repeated. However, the sample size will in general be less since patients with outcome O_2 in the interval $[t, t']$ are dropped from the study. It follows that the coefficients of the risk index (7.3) will differ from those obtained at time t, i.e.,

$$\begin{aligned} I(t') &= a_0(t') + a_1(t')x_1(t') + \cdots + a_k(t')x_k(t') \\ &= a_0(t') + \mathbf{a}^T(t')\mathbf{x}(t') \end{aligned}$$

By applying a variable selection procedure at each time point different subsets of variables may be selected at different times. From this, we could discover when each variable achieves its optimal efficiency in the course of the disease. For example, a variable may be highly significant in the early phase of monitoring, and useless later, or conversely. In addition to allowing variable selection at each time, the repeated logistic method is familiar and relatively simple. It has, of course, the practical disadvantage of producing a different set of coefficients at each time. More importantly, only current measurements are used to compute the index at each time. Thus, the method does not really take the disease process as a whole into account and is "dynamic" only in the sense of being repeated at each time point.

Example: Outcome Prediction After Severe Head Injury

The repeated logistic method was applied to a sample of 61 patients with severe head injury and loss of consciousness admitted to the shock trauma center of Strasbourg, France (Bourguignat et al., 1983)*. Five days after the trauma, 40 patients were still alive. During the first 4 days, specifically at 24, 48, 72, and 96 hours after admission, a laboratory profile of 8 tests was measured: 4 enzymes—aldolase (ALD), aspartate aminotransferase (AST), creatine kinase (CK), and lactate dehydrogenase (LD)—and 4 inflammation markers—α_1-antitrypsin (ANT), fibrinogen (FIB), C-reactive protein (CRP), and leukocytes (WBC). Results were in units of U/L for enzymes, g/L for ANT and FIB, mg/L for CRP, and gigaparticles per liter (G/L) for leukocytes.

In this study, the unit time interval was 24 hours. Since all patients survived at least 5 days, this example does not permit a truly dynamic approach to prognosis. That is, the relative proportions of the different outcomes did not change with time. Nevertheless, repeated application of logistic discrimination did produce some interesting results.

Because of the large number of variables, we first examined the predictive efficiency of each laboratory test separately

---

*This patient sample is entirely distinct from the head injury data (Liège University Hospital) used in Chapter 6, Section 6.4.

TABLE 7.1 Univariate Prognostic Ability of the Eight Laboratory Tests, 24, 48, 72, and 96 Hours After Severe Head Injury[a]

	Time after trauma							
	24 h		48 h		72 h		96 h	
	Test	χ^2	Test	χ^2	Test	χ^2	Test	χ^2
1.	LD	16.80	CRP	24.70	LD	32.86	CRP	40.50
2.	AST	11.80	AST	23.08	CRP	28.44	LD	35.60
3.	WBC	9.98	LD	20.34	WBC	22.78	ANT	28.78
4.	CRP	7.36	WBC	19.52	ANT	22.44	WBC	21.96
5.	CK	6.86	ANT	18.62	ALD	19.68	FIB	19.84
6.	ALD	6.10	ALD	16.06	AST	17.82	AST	16.76
7.	ANT	6.06	CK	12.00	CK	13.32	CK	13.06
8.	FIB	0.15	FIB	11.08	FIB	7.58	ALD	10.00

[a]Results are chi-square values on one degree of freedom observed from applying the logistic model to the set of 61 patients (40 survivors, 21 non-survivors). The chi-square value (1 df) measures the ability of the laboratory test to predict outcome, or in other words, to separate survivors from non-survivors. The chi-square is obtained in exactly the same way as described in Chapter 5.
Source: Bourguignat et al. (1983).

at each time. We then performed stepwise selection at 24, 48, 72, and 96 hours, discarding all redundant variables. The risk index at each time was based on the selected variables only. The efficiency of each constituent at each sampling time is given in Table 7.1. Results correspond to chi-square values with one degree of freedom. Thus, a test significantly discriminates between survivors and nonsurvivors after severe head injury if the chi-square exceeds the critical 5% level, namely 3.84. The laboratory tests are ranked according to decreasing chi-square values, that is, decreasing prognostic efficiency at each time. In all cases but one (FIB at 24 h), the tests are highly significant risk factors. LD and CRP are almost always classified in first or second position, while FIB ranks last. In general, the usefulness of each test increases with time. The maximum value is achieved with CRP at 96 h after trauma (χ^2 = 40.5).

TABLE 7.2 Results of Stepwise Logistic Discrimination Applied to a Sample of 61 Patients (40 Survivors, 21 Nonsurvivors) with Severe Head Injury, Respectively 24, 48, 72, and 96 Hours Later[a]

	Time after trauma							
	24 h		48 hr.		72 h		96 h	
	Test	χ^2	Test	χ^2	Test	χ^2	Test	χ^2
1.	LD	16.80	CRP	24.70	LD	32.86	CRP	40.50
2.	WBC	6.36	ANT	14.20	CRP	13.88	LD	17.76
3.			AST	8.30	WBC	9.12		
4.			WBC	5.98	AST	9.00		
5.			FIB	3.96				

[a]Results are chi-square values on one degree of freedom significant at the 5% critical level.
Source: Data from Bourguignat et al. (1983).

Despite the fact that most variables showed high prognostic efficiency at each sampling time, not all should enter the risk index since correlations exist that make some tests redundant with respect to others. To select the optimal subset of variables, we applied stepwise logistic discriminant analysis at each time point starting always with the best single variable. Results are displayed in Table 7.2. Each figure is a chi-square value on one degree of freedom reflecting the contribution of the variable added to those (above) already selected. The results on the first line are taken from the same line in Table 7.1. Only significant chi-square values are reported in Table 7.2.

We observe that the size and make-up of the vector of selected tests is different at each time. Two variables are sufficient at 24 hours and 96 hours after trauma, while 5 and 4 are needed at 48 hours and 72 hours, respectively. Overall, LD and CRP appear to make important and separate contributions to outcome prediction.

The risk indices based on the daily selected variables were respectively

$$
\begin{aligned}
I\,(24\text{ h}) &= 0.006\text{ LD} + 0.131\text{ WBC} - 4.87 \\
I\,(48\text{ h}) &= 0.010\text{ CRP} + 1.032\text{ ANT} + 0.031\text{ AST} \\
&\quad + 0.271\text{ WBC} - 0.17\text{ FIB} - 9.89 \\
I\,(72\text{ h}) &= 0.017\text{ LD} + 0.097\text{ CRP} \\
&\quad + 0.876\text{ WBC} + 0.052\text{ AST} - 29.56 \\
I\,(96\text{ h}) &= 0.020\text{ LD} + 0.043\text{ CRP} - 11.25
\end{aligned}
$$

These indices can be used to predict eventual outcome in any future patient with severe head injury when the appropriate data become available.

We calculated the four risk indices for each of the 61 patients in the training sample and counted the percentage of correct predictions at each time: they were 77%, 90%, 93.3%, and 93.4%, respectively. Thus, outcome prediction improves with time, achieving its optimal value 4 days after trauma. Although it is of interest to know which variables are clinically useful and when, it is easier from a practical viewpoint to plan measurement of selected variables routinely rather than only at certain sampling times. In the present example, the profile consisting of lactate dehydrogenase and *C*-reactive protein correctly predicted outcome in 68.9%, 78.7%, 85.2%, and 93.4% of the cases after each successive daily sample. These two variables can be regarded as constituting a reasonably satisfactory test profile for monitoring severe head injury.

7.4 EXTENSION OF THE RESPONSE CURVE METHOD

In Chapter 6, we described a method for allocating a patient's response curve $\mathbf{x}(t)$, $a \leq t \leq b$, into one of two groups O_1 and O_2. The basic principle was to calculate the distance between the patient's response curve and the average response curve of each group and then to allocate the patient to the closest group. The distances were calculated over the whole time interval $[a,b]$; thus, allocation was only possible when the response curve was completely observed. In practice, however, one observes a multivariate response curve progressively, as time evolves from a to b. One may therefore wish to apply the classification criterion [equation (6.22)] even with incomplete observation of the response curve $\mathbf{x}(t)$ over $[a,b]$.

As before, let $\bar{\mathbf{x}}_1(t)$ and $\bar{\mathbf{x}}_2(t)$, $a \leq t \leq b$, be the average response curves in outcome groups O_1 and O_2, respectively. Suppose that the response curve $\mathbf{x}(t)$ for a new patient has been observed only until time t ($t \leq b$). Then the distances between $\mathbf{x}(t)$ and the two average curves over the interval $[a, t]$ are given by ($j = 1, 2$):

$$D_t^2(\mathbf{x},\bar{\mathbf{x}}_j) = (t-a)^{-1} \int_a^t \{\mathbf{x}(t') - \bar{\mathbf{x}}_j(t')\}^T \mathbf{S}^{-1}(t') \{\mathbf{x}(t') - \bar{\mathbf{x}}_j(t')\} dt' \qquad (7.5)$$

The suffix t for the distance indicates that the distance between the two response curves is calculated from the fixed origin a to the varying endpoint t.

All the mathematical developments in Section 6.6 apply when distance (7.5) is used instead of distance (6.15), and after some simplifications (Albert, 1983), the risk index (6.22) becomes

$$I_t(\mathbf{x}) = (t-a)^{-1} \operatorname{tr}\{\mathbf{C}_t(\mathbf{A}^T\mathbf{Y}_t + \mathbf{B})\} \qquad (7.6)$$

where the matrices $\mathbf{A}$ and $\mathbf{B}$ are given by equations (6.23). The matrix $\mathbf{Y}_t$ is a $k \times q$ matrix containing all the observations available at time t (the elements not yet observed are replaced by zeroes), and the matrix $\mathbf{C}_t$ is defined as in Section 6.6 but with all elements corresponding to $t_i \geq t$ set to zero. The equation (7.6) defines a time-dependent risk index that can be calculated for each time point t. When $t = b$, we retrieve exactly the same value as with the static index (6.22). So the dynamic risk index provides at each time the relative location of the patient with respect to the two outcome groups O_1 and O_2.

Application to Continuous Risk Assessment After Acute MI

Let us reconsider the acute myocardial infarction prognostic problem discussed in Section 6.7. A 70-year-old man with no previous infarcts is admitted to the coronary care unit with documented MI. Daily laboratory data are given in Table 6.3. We shall now attempt to predict the patient's status during the 24 hours following each day's vector of laboratory data. At admission, the patient's laboratory profile is: urea = 0.45 g/L and LD = 500 U/L. The matrix $\mathbf{Y}_t$ at $t = 0$ consists of the first column of Table 6.3 with all other columns set equal to zero. Likewise, matrix $\mathbf{C}_t$ has all elements zero except for unity at the intersection of the first row and first column. Using the matrices **A** and **B** given in Tables 6.7 and 6.8, and substituting all these quantities into equation (7.6), we find $I_0(\mathbf{x}) = -0.31$. Note that when $t = a$ in equation (7.6), the factor $(t - a)$ is replaced by 1.

On the first day after admission, the patient's laboratory values are: urea = 0.48 g/L and LD = 2238 U/L, and proceeding as above, his index becomes $I_1(\mathbf{x}) = +0.27$. The patient has crossed the zero cutoff point and enters the positive, unfavorable zone. This is mainly due to the elevation of LD. The index score $I_1(\mathbf{x})$ assesses the patient's risk with respect to death and survival on the basis of the response curve from admission to day 1.

The same procedure can be repeated for the subsequent days. All results for this patient are displayed in Figure 7.1. From the time of admission the patient's score climbs more and more into the unfavorable zone. This reflects the high urea and LD concentrations throughout hospitalization. On day 6, the risk index is equal to 2.88, the value found in Section 6.7. This final score is based on the entire response curve from admission to day 6, not solely on the results that day.

Further examples of the application of the response curve method to laboratory data can be found in Albert et al. (1982) and in Chapelle et al. (1983).

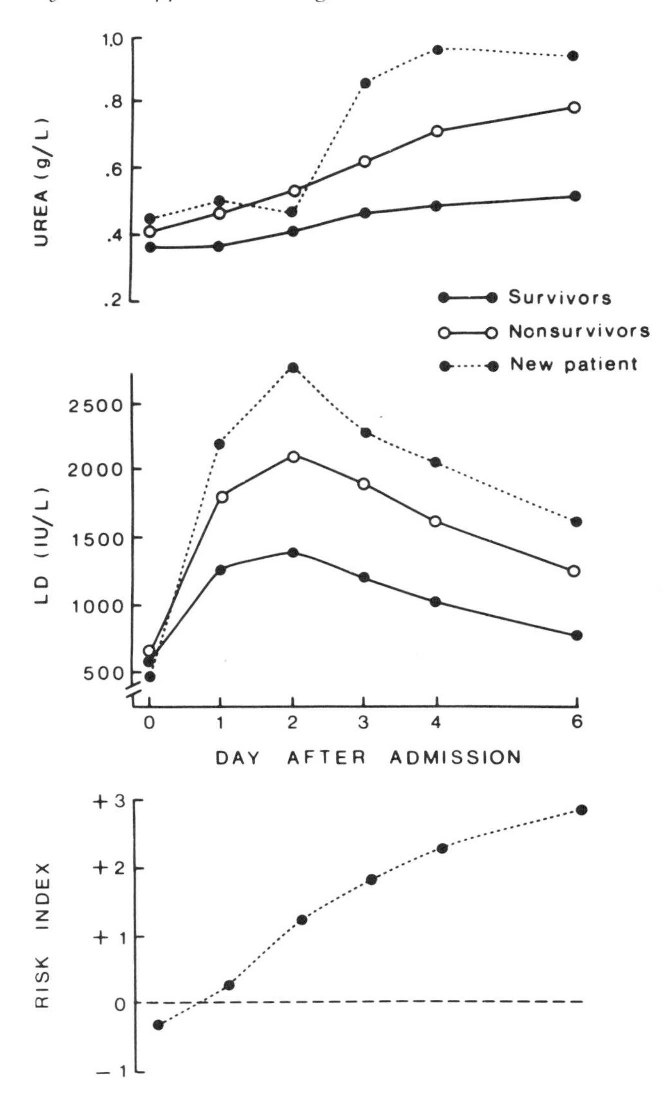

FIGURE 7.1 Application of the response curve method to calculate the dynamic risk index based on urea (g/L) and LD (U/L) concentrations for a 70-year-old MI patient with no previous infarct. Average response curves for survivors (n = 120) and nonsurvivors (n = 12) are represented by solid lines, while the patient's evolution is shown by dotted lines. Positive values of the risk index are signs of unfavorable evolution (Albert, 1983).

The response curve approach is purely descriptive, but, unlike the repeated discriminant analysis described in Section 7.3, it does take into account the biochemical process as a whole. However, as mentioned in Chapter 6, it does not allow full scope to the selection of variables, except through Zerbe's univariate F-tests. It does not, at present, permit statistical testing of significance of a risk index and calculation of posterior probabilities. Moreover, we are still constrained under equation (7.6) as under equation (6.22) to include in the training sample only those patients who survived at least through to the end of the monitoring period (i.e., through $t = b$).

To preserve the good points of the two methods so far discussed while overcoming their faults, we describe in the next section a better method for dynamic outcome prediction. This method can be viewed as the direct extension of logistic discrimination to time-dependent observations and outcome. Therefore, it may be expected to have similar properties of simplicity, generality, and robustness.

7.5 EXTENSION OF THE LOGISTIC MODEL TO TIME-RELATED DATA

A. Definition of the Dynamic Risk Index

Assuming that patients are monitored at regular time intervals, let us now address the statistical problem described in Section 7.2: to predict the patient's outcome Y_t in the next unit time interval from *past* data, $\mathbf{U}^T = \{\mathbf{x}^T(t), \mathbf{x}^T(t - 1), \ldots\}$. It is clear that we are free to decide what we should consider as the past. At one extreme, it may consist solely of the baseline variables; at another, it contains all baseline and time-dependent data available for the patient at time t. In most situations, reliable prediction can be achieved at each time using only limited information collected from the patient.

We want a model to compute the posterior probability of each outcome in the next time interval from the past of the patient, i.e., $\text{pr}(y_t = 1|\mathbf{U}_t)$ and $\text{pr}(y_t = 2|\mathbf{U}_t)$, and to repeat the calculation whenever the next observation becomes available. In contrast to the classical situation, both the outcome variable Y_t and the vector of covariates $\mathbf{U}_t$ depend on the time factor t.

The direct extension (Wu and Ware, 1979) of the classical logistic model described in Section 6.2 to time-dependent outcome and predictors is given by the following model ($t = 0, 1, \ldots$):

$$\text{pr}(y_t = 2|\mathbf{U}_t) = \frac{\exp\{I(t)\}}{1 + \exp\{I(t)\}} \tag{7.7}$$

where the function

$$\begin{aligned} I(t) &= a_0(t) + \mathbf{a}_1^T(t)\mathbf{x}(t) + \mathbf{a}_2^T(t)\mathbf{x}(t-1) + \cdots \\ &= a_0(t) + \mathbf{a}^T(t)\mathbf{U}_t \end{aligned} \tag{7.8}$$

is a linear combination of past observations at time t. Equation (7.8) defines a dynamic risk index, calculable at all times. Equation (7.7) simply states that the posterior probability of death in the interval $[t, t + 1]$ is a logistic function of the dynamic risk index $I(t)$.

As in the classical approach, the unknowns in this model are the intercept $a_0(t)$ and the vector of weighting factors $\mathbf{a}^T(t) = \{\mathbf{a}_1^T(t), \mathbf{a}_2^T(t), \ldots\}$. In general, however, these parameters are themselves time dependent and have to be estimated from the data at each time. The model is then said to be nonstationary. The assumption of constant weights over time (stationary model) would considerably simplify the model and the estimation problem; unfortunately, it is unrealistic in many acute disease situations. To solve this problem, a single variable transform (Albert et al., 1984b) has been suggested.

B. Variable Transform and Stationary Model

It is proposed to transform the vector of covariates $\mathbf{U}_t$ in such a way that for the new vector, say $\mathbf{Z}_t$, a stationary model is applicable. Then,

$$\begin{aligned} I(t) &= b_0 + \mathbf{b}_1^T\mathbf{z}(t) + \mathbf{b}_2^T\mathbf{z}(t-1) + \cdots \\ &= b_0 + \mathbf{b}^T\mathbf{Z}_t \qquad (t = 0,1, \ldots) \end{aligned} \tag{7.9}$$

and

$$P_t = \text{pr}(y_t = 2|\mathbf{Z}_t) = \frac{\exp\{I(t)\}}{1 + \exp\{I(t)\}} \tag{7.10}$$

where b_0 and $\mathbf{b}^T = (\mathbf{b}_1^T, \mathbf{b}_2^T, \ldots)$ are a set of unknown parameters, no longer time dependent. The dynamic risk index $I(t)$ remains a function of time only through the transformed vector $\mathbf{Z}_t$.

To achieve this stationarity, we observe that in many diseases where there is an acute phase, serial laboratory data collected from the patients follow a deterministic pattern. For example, after an acute myocardial infarction, there is a typical rise and fall of serum cardiac enzymes. Likewise in severe head injury, inflammation markers tend to deplete after a marked elevation. The patterns of change in both survivors and nonsurvivors are generally similar in shape but differ in size, the latter usually exhibiting higher test results as an indication of poor prognosis. Thus, if we subtract the deterministic component from all individual response curves, our choice being the average response curve for survivors, we are left with data that fluctuate around the zero baseline for survivors and around some positive threshold value for nonsurvivors. For example, consider the average response curves of lactate dehydrogenase in survivors of MI and suppose we have observed the LD values in a new myocardial infarction patient. To subtract the deterministic component from the observed

LD response curve, it suffices to standardize the observed value at each time by computing $z = (x - \bar{x})/SD$. If on day 2 after admission, the mean and standard deviation of LD in known survivors of MI are 1418 U/L and 623 U/L, respectively, and the LD value observed in the new patient is 2300 U/L, then the standardized value at that time becomes $z = (2300 - 1418)/623 = +1.42$.

If all time-dependent variables are transformed as described (there being no need to apply such a transformation to baseline variables), the assumption of a stationary model given by equations (7.9) and (7.10) can be considered reasonable for describing the prognostic situation. The problem is then reduced to estimating the intercept b_0 and the vector of coefficients **b**.

C. Estimation of the Parameters of the Dynamic Risk Index

To estimate all unknown coefficients appearing in the dynamic risk index [equation (7.9)], it is assumed that data from a sample of n patients have been recorded at regular times (e.g., daily) during a specified monitoring period (e.g., one week), and that their outcome (alive or deceased) is also known in every interval of time. Let τ denote the last time interval during which observations were recorded. Estimates of the unknown parameters b_0 and **b** are obtained by maximizing the log-likelihood function of the sample denoted by $\log L$. By definition,

$$\log L(b_0, \mathbf{b}) = \sum_{t=1}^{\tau} \sum_{j=1}^{2} \sum_{i \in E_{tj}} \log P_{ijt} \tag{7.11}$$

where E_{tj} is the set of all patients having outcome j in the t-th interval of time, and $P_{ijt} = \text{pr}(y_{ti} = j|\mathbf{Z}_{ti})$ represents the probability that the ith patient has outcome j in the t-th interval given his or her "past" vector $\mathbf{Z}_{ti}$. In equation (7.11), the P_{ijt} terms are replaced by

$$P_{ijt} = \frac{\exp(b_0 + \mathbf{b}^T\mathbf{Z}_{ti})}{1 + \exp(b_0 + \mathbf{b}^T\mathbf{Z}_{ti})} \tag{7.12}$$

if the patient has outcome $j = 2$ in the t-th interval of time and the complementary expression $\{1 + \exp(b_0 + \mathbf{b}^T\mathbf{Z}_{ti})\}^{-1}$ if $j = 1$.

The maximization of (7.11) with respect to b_0 and $\mathbf{b}$ is performed using the well-known Newton-Raphson iterative procedure.

7.6 SELECTING THE APPROPRIATE INFORMATION FOR THE DYNAMIC RISK INDEX

When trying to derive an optimal dynamic risk index, two questions arise: (1) Which variables (baseline and time-dependent) should enter the index; and (2) for time-dependent variables, how many past observations are required to achieve satisfactory prediction? To answer these questions, we proceed by considering models of increasing complexity. That is, we maximize the function (7.11) for different models of the posterior probabilities P_{ijt}. Since the vector $\mathbf{Z}_t$ contains all the past information available at time t, we are free to decide what should be included in this vector.

A. The One-Parameter Model M_1

The simplest model (M_1) is to say that $\mathbf{Z}_t$ is empty, i.e., that the patient has lived up to time t but no past observations are available. Surely this is unrealistic, but it provides a start. In this case, equation (7.9) reduced to $I(t) = b_0$, a constant. The risk index associated with every patient is then the same at all times. Further, the posterior probability (7.10) becomes

$$P_t = \frac{\exp(b_0)}{1 + \exp(b_0)} \tag{7.13}$$

P_t is called the "hazard function" (Kalbfleisch and Prentice,

1980; Cox and Oakes, 1984), which in this particular case is also a constant p_0, say. It represents the immediate risk of death, i.e., the probability of dying in the next unit time interval given that the patient has survived up to time t. The value of b_0 may be obtained by maximizing the log likelihood function (7.11) which under model M_1 reduces to

$$\log L(b_0) = \sum_{t=1}^{T} \{n_{t1} \log (1 - p_0) + n_{t2} \log (p_0)\} \tag{7.14}$$

where n_{t1} and n_{t2} are the number of subjects with outcome $y_t = 1$ and $y_t = 2$ in the t-th interval of time and $p_0 = \exp(b_0)/\{1 + \exp(b_0)\}$. The maximum likelihood estimate of b_0 in this simple model is that value for which p_0 equals the average observed death rate during a unit time interval.

B. The Two-Parameter Model M_2

Another simple model assumes that the past vector $\mathbf{Z}_t$ contains only a baseline variable, say z. The risk index (7.9) becomes $I(t) = b_0 + b_1 z$, which again does not depend on time. However, in contrast to model M_1, the value of $I(t)$ is different for every patient, since z changes from one subject to another (e.g., z = age of patient).

The hazard function

$$P_t = \frac{\exp(b_0 + b_1 z)}{1 + \exp(b_0 + b_1 z)} \tag{7.15}$$

is still a constant but varies with the values of z. It represents the immediate risk of death given that the patient has survived until time t and his or her baseline variable equals z. Estimates of b_0 and b_1, the two parameters of the model, are obtained by maximizing equation (7.11) where expression (7.15) is substituted for the P_{ijt} terms. For example, in the acute myocardial infarction data described below, the average daily risk of death p_0 is 1.5%, but increases to 3.3% for a 70-year-old patient.

If instead of adding a baseline variable to model M_1, we use the most recent observation $z(t)$ of any time-dependent variable, we still have a two-parameter model, but the risk index (7.9) becomes

$$I(t) = b_0 + b_1 z(t) \tag{7.16}$$

a time-dependent function. Likewise the hazard function

$$P_t = \frac{\exp\{b_0 + b_1 z(t)\}}{1 + \exp\{b_0 + b_1 z(t)\}} \tag{7.17}$$

varies with time as well as with each individual. Here we really start modeling each patient's particular evolution. The value of P_t can rise or fall depending on the value of the (biochemical) variable Z.

The estimates b_0 and b_1 are again obtained by maximizing (7.11), into which the expression (7.17) has been inserted.

C. The Three-Parameter Model M_3

Three-parameter models are obtained by looking at the combination of two variables. Several possibilities can be envisaged. The past vector $\mathbf{Z}_t$ contains:

1. Two baseline variables z_1 and z_2

$$I(t) = b_0 + b_1 z_1 + b_2 z_2$$

2. One baseline variable and the most recent observation of a time-dependent variable

$$I(t) = b_0 + b_1 z_1 + b_2 z_2(t)$$

3. The most recent observation of two time-dependent variables

$$I(t) = b_0 + b_1 z_1(t) + b_2 z_2(t)$$

4. The last two observations of a time-dependent variable

$$I(t) = b_0 + b_1 z_1(t) + b_2 z_2(t - 1)$$

This last model would be used to test whether the previous observation of the variable significantly improves the outcome prediction based on the most recent observation.

D. More General Models

Proceeding as above, we can design more complicated expressions to model the risk index and the hazard function. In fact, we may look at any combination of data collected from the patients. An extremely large number of possibilities exists if many variables are studied and time points considered. The most complete model, given by equations (7.9) and (7.10), involves the entire past record of the patient's observations.

E. Selection Criteria

Given the numerous possible associations of variables, the following stepwise manner is recommended:

Step 1: Fit the one-parameter model: $I(t) = b_0$.

Step 2: Fit the two-parameter model: $I(t) = b_0 + b_1 z$, where z is any baseline variable, or any time-dependent variable measured at time t.

Step 3: Choose the best two-parameter model, denote the variable selected by z_1, and fit the three-parameter model $I(t) = b_0 + b_1 z_1 + b_2 z$ for any possible z as described in step 2.

Step 4: Carry on the selection procedure as stated in step 2 (i.e., variables measured at time t), until there is no significant improvement in prediction when adding the remaining variables.

Step 5: Test in a similar way whether previous observations (time $t - 1, t - 2, \ldots$) for any time-dependent variable improve the efficiency of the dynamic risk index.

This procedure is not always feasible when the number of possible combinations is large. The user may then determine on the basis of previous experience and knowledge the order in which the data should enter the dynamic index. This should speed up the selection process. To test whether added data significantly improve the efficiency of the risk index, one may use a log-likelihood ratio criterion asymptotically distributed as a χ^2-variable on one degree of freedom. If $\log L_k$ and $\log L_{k+1}$ denote the maximized log-likelihoods when k and $k + 1$ variables are respectively included in the index $I(t)$, then the variable added is selected if the criterion

$$2(\log L_{k+1} - \log L_k) \tag{7.18}$$

exceeds the upper 5% critical point of the chi-square distribution on one degree of freedom.

This criterion can only be applied if the two models M_k and M_{k+1} are embedded in a hierarchy. This means that all variables in model M_k must also be in model M_{k+1}. One possible approach to the comparison of models with different variables is to compute for each model Akaike's Information Criterion,

$$\text{AIC} = -2 \log \hat{L} + 2\nu \tag{7.19}$$

where $\log \hat{L}$ is the maximized log-likelihood and ν the number of estimated parameters. The "best" model is the one for which AIC is a minimum.

7.7
EFFICIENCY OF THE DYNAMIC RISK INDEX

Suppose that an "optimal" dynamic risk index has been derived. It is not easy to measure the efficiency of this index, because in addition to the multivariate aspect of the problem, a time factor is involved. In the "static" situation, efficiency is determined by recalculating the index for all patients and counting the number of patients correctly classified. In the present context, we need to look at prediction on a day-to-day basis. One possible solution is to compute the dynamic index $I(t)$ for all patients of the database (or of a validation sample) at all time intervals ($t = 1, \ldots, \tau$); for nonsurvivors, the index is calculated until death. If for each patient we select the worst score I_w over the entire monitoring period (or until death), we can examine the distributions of this score in the two groups, survivors and nonsurvivors, and determine the cutoff point I_w^* where these distributions intersect (see Chapter 4). If we define the specificity of the index $I(t)$ as the proportion of survivors with a score $I_w \leq I_w^*$, and the sensitivity as the proportion of nonsurvivors with $I_w > I_w^*$, these values can be used to indicate the efficiency of the method.

Another way to measure the performance of the index consists of calculating for each patient the "accumulated conditional probability of death" given by the equation

$$\pi = P_1 + \sum_{t=2}^{\tau} P_t \prod_{t'=1}^{t-1} (1 - P_{t'}) \tag{7.20}$$

where P_t is the probability of death in the t-th interval as given by equation (7.10) and τ the last interval for which the patient was still alive. The value of π represents the overall posterior probability of death of the patient during the monitoring period, based on a predictive model which includes at each time point a specified amount of past information. We would expect that survivors yield low values for π, and nonsurvivors high values. Again, differences between the distributions of these accumulated probabilities for survivors and nonsurvivors may provide interesting information about the efficiency of the dynamic risk index $I(t)$.

7.8
INDIVIDUAL INTERPRETATION OF THE DYNAMIC INDEX

The prior probability of death in any patient is equal to p_0, the average observed death rate in a unit time interval. Under model M_1, $p_0 = \exp(b_0)/\{1 + \exp(b_0)\}$. At time t, knowledge of the patient's past record yields a risk index $I(t)$ and a posterior probability P_t of dying in the next interval of time. Thus the ratio

$$R_t = \frac{P_t}{p_0} \qquad (t = 1,2, \ldots) \tag{7.21}$$

indicates how much the prior probability has changed given the observations up to time t recorded on this particular patient. At any time, a value of R_t below 1 is a sign of a favorable evolution, while a value of R_t above 1 indicates an increase of risk above the average.

7.9
APPLICATION TO ACUTE MYOCARDIAL INFARCTION

To illustrate the methodology described in Sections 7.5 to 7.8, we applied it to 330 myocardial infarction patients, diagnosed on the basis of typical clinical history, electrocardiographic evidence and serum enzyme changes (Albert et al., 1984a). The patient's age and number of previous episodes of myocardial infarction, denoted by nMI, were also recorded on

TABLE 7.3 Mortality Rate During the First Week of Hospitalization for the Sample of 330 Patients with Acute Myocardial Infarction

Day after admission	Number of daily deaths	Cumulative mortality rate (%)
1	3	0.9
2	5	2.4
3	8	4.8
4	3	5.8
5	2	6.3
6	4	7.6
7	8	10.0

Source: Chapelle et al. (1984).

admission for every patient. The mean age was 57.4 (SD = 9.5) years; 65 patients (19.7%) had a prior history of myocardial infarction. The day-to-day distribution of deaths from cardiac causes during the investigation period is shown in Table 7.3; 33 patients died during this period, leading to an overall mortality rate of 10%. The average daily death rate among the survivors to the beginning of each day was p_0 = 0.015, or 1.5%.

For each patient, seven serum biochemical parameters were measured daily for one week: creatine kinase (CK, U/L); lactate dehydrogenase (LD, U/L); α_1-acid glycoprotein (AGP, g/L); haptoglobin (Hp, g/L); uric acid (UA, mg/L); urea (g/L); and creatinine (CR, mg/L).

A. Transformation of the Time-Dependent Observations

The average evolution of each biochemical parameter in the one-year survivor group was considered as the "standard" response curve and constituted the deterministic component to which we referred in Section 7.5(B). In order to use the

TABLE 7.4 Daily Means and Standard Deviations (SD) of Seven Serum Constituents During the First Week of Acute Hospitalization Obtained from 272 One-Year Myocardial Infarction Survivors

	Day after admission						
Variables	0	1	2	3	4	5	6
CK (U/L)	326	1134	479	226	161	124	87
	(434)	(810)	(450)	(265)	(197)	(135)	(101)
LD (U/L)	571	1323	1418	1249	1031	916	800
	(292)	(570)	(623)	(542)	(412)	(344)	(291)
AGP (g/L)	0.90	1.07	1.34	1.50	1.58	1.60	1.63
	(0.21)	(0.31)	(0.28)	(0.33)	(0.38)	(0.40)	(0.43)
Hp (g/L)	2.27	2.81	3.68	4.23	4.56	4.67	4.78
	(0.97)	(1.27)	(1.47)	(1.47)	(1.57)	(1.58)	(1.65)
UA (mg/L)	61.9	57.5	56.6	58.1	60.6	61.4	62.2
	(13.7)	(14.0)	(14.9)	(15.5)	(15.9)	(15.7)	(16.4)
Urea (g/L)	0.38	0.37	0.40	0.45	0.48	0.49	0.50
	(0.13)	(0.16)	(0.18)	(0.20)	(0.21)	(0.21)	(0.23)
CR (mg/L)	10.8	10.9	11.2	11.4	11.4	11.4	11.5
	(3.3)	(3.4)	(3.7)	(4.0)	(4.1)	(4.1)	(4.4)

Source: Chapelle et al. (1984).

stationary model [equation (7.7)] for which the coefficients are constant over the monitoring period, we "standardized" (i.e., transformed each observation x to $z = (x - \bar{x})/SD$, using the corresponding daily means and standard deviations (SD) for one-year survivors given in Table 7.4. As an example of the transformation, we compared the LD activities serially recorded during one week for a particular patient with the "standard" evolution of this enzyme in the survivor group (see Figure 7.2). The lower part of the diagram displays the evolution of the reduced variable z. For instance, on day 2 after admission, the LD activities measured for the patient and for the one-year survivors (see Table 7.4) are 1950 and 1418 U/L ($SD = 623$), respectively, so that the corrected value becomes $z = (1950 - 1418)/623 = +0.85$. Note that a negative value of z was observed on day 1 because the LD activity recorded for the patient was lower than that of the "standard" curve.

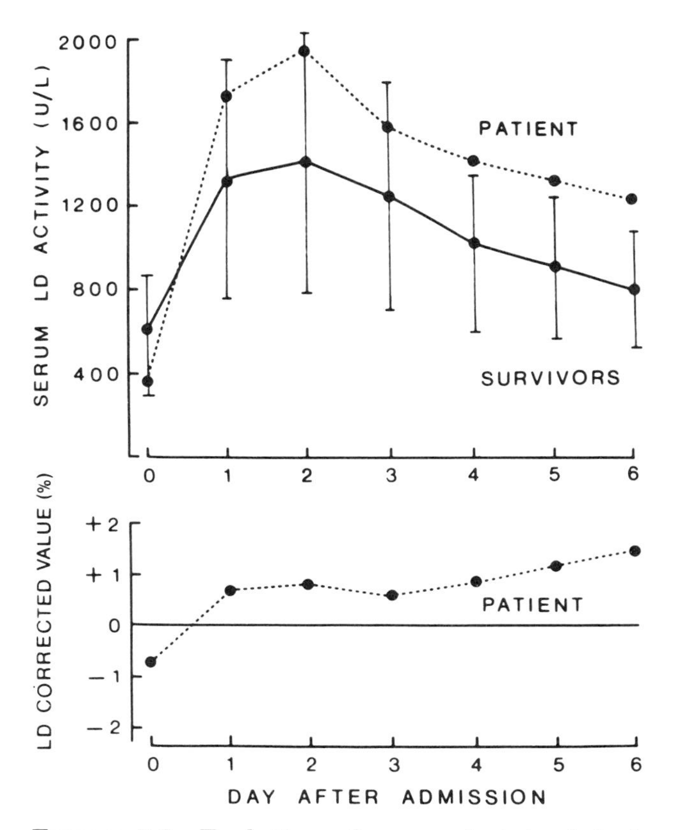

FIGURE 7.2 Evolution of serum lactate dehydrogenase activity during the first week after a myocardial infarction for one-year survivors and for a new MI patient. The lower part of the diagram displays the patient's LD-values after standardization as described in the text (Chapelle et al., 1984).

B. Fitting the Model M_1: Prior Hazard Function

Under model M_1, for which $p_0 = \exp(b_0)/\{1 + \exp(b_0)\}$, the maximum likelihood estimate of b_0 is -4.18. It follows that the hazard function is $p_0 = 0.015$, which, as noted earlier, corresponds to the average daily death rate. The quantity $p_0 = 0.015$ enables us to calculate other probabilities under this model. For instance, the probability of dying within the four first days of hospitalization is equal to $0.015 + (0.985)(0.015) + (0.985)^2(0.015) + (0.985)^3(0.015) = 0.044$. However, the observed proportions of nonsurvivors after four days (see Table 7.3) was 0.058.

C. Fitting the Two-Parameter Model

The univariate dynamic predictive power of each variable was determined by fitting to the data a two-parameter model involving only the most recent observation $z(t)$ of a time-dependent variable or the baseline values:

$$I(t) = b_0 + b_1 z(t) \tag{7.22}$$

This model was compared with the simplest model M_1 using the chi-square criterion (7.18). The biochemical variables were ordered according to decreasing efficiency (see Table 7.5, column 2). The chi-square values obtained show that LD and urea are the best risk predictors, whereas AGP appears to have the least usefulness for day-to-day prognostication. The predictive values for creatinine, CK, uric acid, and haptoglobin are intermediate. As all chi-square results were significant at the 5% level, we concluded that there exists, for each biochemical parameter investigated, a relationship between the most recently observed serum concentration or activity and the outcome occurring on the following day; this relationship, however, decreases steeply from LD to AGP. The two baseline variables, age on admission ($\chi^2 = 15.6$) and the number of previous myocardial infarctions ($\chi^2 = 4.1$), were significant risk factors.

D. Fitting Other Models

We investigated other models of outcome prediction by combining two or several variables together. We first fitted the model

TABLE 7.5 Univariate Dynamic Prognostic Efficiency of the Variables Investigated (Chi-Square Test, 1 df)[a]; Effect of Previous Measurements for Each Time-dependent Variable; the Chi-Square Values Are Obtained by Comparing Models (7.22) and (7.24)

Variable	Efficiency of result of day t (χ^2 on 1 df)[b]	Effect of result of day $t-1$ (χ^2 on 1 df)
Time-dependent:		
1. LD	47.06	0.74 N.S.
2. Urea	41.82	1.36 N.S.
3. Creatinine	16.82	2.80 N.S.
4. CK	16.70	5.86 $p < 0.05$
5. Uric acid	14.65	16.64 $p < 0.01$
6. Hp	13.44	3.10 N.S.
7. AGP	4.42	0.42 N.S.
Baseline:		
8. Age	15.59	
9. nMI	4.06	

[a]Variables are listed according to decreasing chi-square values.
[b]All χ^2 values are significant at the 5% critical level.
Source: Chapelle et al. (1984).

$$I(t) = b_0 + b_1 \text{age} + b_2 nMI + b_3 z(t) \tag{7.23}$$

where $z(t)$ denotes the most recent observation of any of the time-dependent variables. We found that the best improvement in prediction was obtained with LD ($\chi^2 = 37.3, p < 0.001$). Next, the value recorded on day t for each remaining variable was successively tested in conjunction with the triplet "age, nMI, and LD(t)." Only urea(t) significantly improved the prediction ($\chi^2 = 21.4$, $p < 0.001$). Consequently, all the other variables were considered to be without prognostic importance when combined with LD and urea, and they were not included in the dynamic index.

To assess the usefulness of previous measurements on outcome prediction, we fitted the three-parameter model

$$I(t) = b_0 + b_1 z(t) + b_2 z(t - 1) \quad (7.24)$$

where $z(t - 1)$ and $z(t)$, respectively, represent the standardized values of the biochemical variable measured on days $t - 1$ and t. The improvement in prediction was assessed by a chi-square test on one degree of freedom obtained by comparing model (7.24) above with model (7.22), which considered only the latest measurement. Results are given in column 3 of Table 7.5. A positive effect of the next most recent observation on outcome prediction was observed for uric acid ($\chi^2 = 16.6$) and CK ($\chi^2 = 5.9$). An explanation for this result on pathophysiologic grounds is given in Chapelle et al. (1984). Since no significant values were obtained for LD and urea, only the most recent measurements of these two variables are of prognostic value.

E. Derivation of the Dynamic Risk Index

From the preceding considerations, we derived a dynamic index based on four covariates: the two baseline variables, age and *nMI*, and the most recent observations of LD and urea. We verified that previous values of uric acid and CK did not result in a significant difference when added to the four factors selected. The final equation of the dynamic prognostic index was:

$$I(t) = 0.038 \text{ age} + 0.58\, nMI + 0.38\, u(t) + 0.31\, L(t) - 7.14 \quad (7.25)$$

Note that, in equation (7.25), $u(t)$ and $L(t)$ represent the standardized values of urea and LD at time t. As mentioned previously, these transformed values depend on the values calculated at the same time for one-year survivors. Table 7.6 illustrates the use of the method for a 62-year-old patient without previous history of myocardial infarction ($nMI = 0$). Corrected values of urea and LD levels recorded during the first week of hospitalization were easily obtained using the

TABLE 7.6 Application of the Dynamic Risk Index Method to a Patient with Acute Myocardial Infarction[a]

Time after admission (days)	Urea levels (g/L)	LD activities (U/L)	Standardized values		Index value [I(t)]	Probability death (P_t)	Risk ratio[b] (R_t)
			Urea	LD			
0	0.25	350	−1.00	−0.75	−5.40	0.0045	0.30
1	0.25	1728	−0.75	0.71	−4.85	0.0078	0.51
2	0.25	1950	−0.83	0.85	−4.84	0.0079	0.52
3	0.27	1569	−0.90	0.59	−4.94	0.0070	0.47
4	0.34	1404	−0.66	0.90	−4.76	0.0085	0.57
5	0.56	1321	0.33	1.17	−4.29	0.0134	0.90
6	0.79	1238	1.26	1.50	−3.84	0.0210	1.40

[a]Aged 62, with no previous infarct (nMI = 0), who died 15 days after his admission to the coronary care unit.
[b]Assuming a constant daily death rate of 1.5%.
Source: Chapelle et al. (1984).

data in Table 7.4. Urea rose from −1.00 to 1.26, and LD from −0.75 to 1.50, indicating a worsening in the evolution of these two parameters as time elapsed. Using equation (7.25), we found that the risk index increased from −5.40 on admission to −3.84 at the end of the first week. This pessimistic trend was confirmed by the daily probabilities of death P_t, as calculated from equation (7.10). Likewise, the risk ratios, $R_t = P_t/p_0$, where $p_0 = 0.015$, increased almost fivefold within one week. Actually, the patient died 15 days after the acute event and this outcome could have been suggested by the data collected during the first week.

F. Efficiency of the Dynamic Risk Index

The global efficiency of the risk index was appraised by computing the index for every patient of the database at all times, and then selecting for survivors the worst of the seven index scores and for nonsurvivors the last index preceding death.

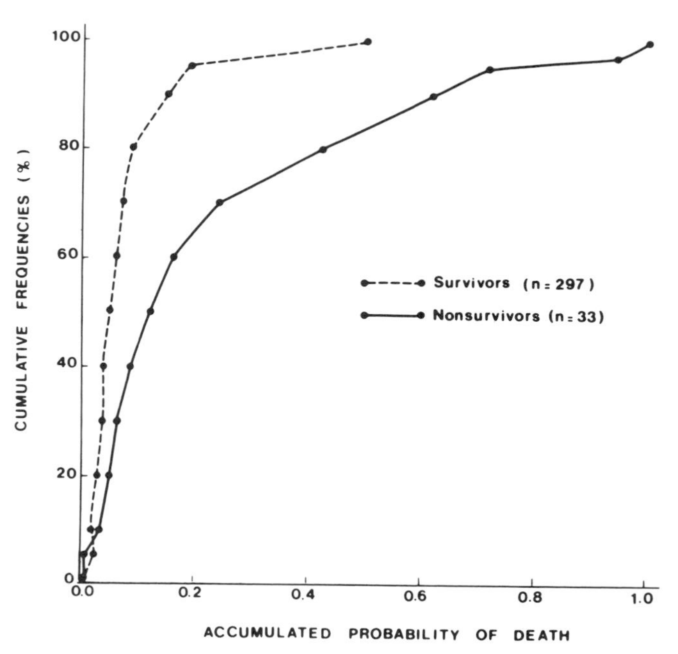

Figure 7.3 Cumulative frequency distributions of the accumulated conditional probability of death (π) in survivor and nonsurvivor groups (Albert et al., 1984b).

The distributions of these scores for survivors and nonsurvivors intersected at a cutoff point of -3.88, i.e., at a value equally likely for both groups. Using this cutoff point for predicting the patient's outcome, we found that 80% of survivors and 72% of nonsurvivors were correctly classified. When using age and *nMI* only, the percentages of correct allocation were 67% and 58%, respectively, emphasizing the usefulness of daily LD and urea results. Further, as Figure 7.3 reveals, the cumulative frequency distributions of the accumulated probabilities of death [equation (7.20)] in survivors ($n = 297$) and in nonsurvivors ($n = 33$) are notably distinct, thus verifying the prognostic value of the index (7.25).

REFERENCES

Albert, A. (1983). Discriminant analysis based on multivariate response curves: A descriptive approach to dynamic allocation. *Stat. Med. 2*, 95–106.

Albert, A., Chapelle, J. P., and Bourguignat, A. (1984a). Dynamic outcome prediction from repeated measurements made on intensive care unit patients. I. Statistical aspects and logistic models. *Scand. J. Clin. Lab. Invest. 44, suppl. 171*, 259–268.

Albert, A., Chapelle, J. P., Heusghem, C., Kulbertus, H. E., and Harris, E. K. (1982). Evaluation of risk using serial laboratory data in acute myocardial infarction. In *Advanced Interpretation of Clinical Laboratory Data,* C. Heusghem, A. Albert, and E. S. Benson (Eds.), Marcel Dekker, New York, pp. 117–130.

Albert, A., Harris, E. K., Chapelle, J. P., Heusghem, C., and Kulbertus, H. E. (1984b). On the interpretation of serial laboratoratory measurements in acute myocardial infarction. *Clin. Chem. 30*, 69–76.

Bourguignat, A., Albert, A., Férard, G., Tulasne, P. A., Kempf, I., and Métais, P. (1983). Prognostic value of combined data on enzymes and inflammation markers in plasma in cases of severe head injury. *Clin. Chem. 29*, 1904–1907.

Chapelle, J. P., Albert, A., and Bourguignat, A. (1984). Dynamic outcome prediction from repeated measurements made on intensive care unit patients. II. Application to acute myocardial infarction. *Scand. J. Clin. Lab. Invest. 44, Suppl. 171*, 269–278.

Chapelle, J. P., Albert, A., Kulbertus, H. E., and Heusghem, C. (1983). The long-term prognostic significance of biochemical measurements obtained during the acute phase of myocardial infarction. In *The First Year After a Myocardial Infarction,* H. E. Kulbertus and H. J. J. Wellens (Eds.). Futura Publishing Company, New York, pp. 15–26.

Cox, D. R., and Oakes, D. (1984). Analysis of Survival Data. Chapman and Hall, London.

Kalbfleisch, J. D., and Prentice, R. L. (1980). *The Statistical Analysis of Failure Time Data.* Wiley, New York.

Wu, M. C., and Ware, J. H. (1979). On the use of repeated measurements in regression analysis with dichotomous responses. *Biometrics 35*, 513–521.

8

TIME SERIES FOR PATIENT MONITORING

8.1 INTRODUCTION

In this chapter, we shall continue our analysis of laboratory results over time but with a different type of patient in mind. The patient now is assumed to be in a more or less "steady state." For example, he or she may fit one of the following descriptions: (i) a healthy individual, pursuing regular daily activities but appearing periodically for a physical checkup, including a battery of blood tests; (ii) an outpatient on prescribed medication following diagnosis and treatment in the hospital; (iii) an inpatient, perhaps in post-operative care, being monitored for signs of possible complications. In any case, the clinician does not expect to see any systematic changes in serial test results but is alert to that possibility and the need for timely intervention to return the patient to the desired state.

With this new type of patient, we shall be introducing a fundamentally different kind of statistical analysis. Up until now, the statistical formulas used to predict the future of a given patient have been based on information obtained from a reference or "training" set of individuals. Of course, such predictions also take account of measurements made on the particular patient involved, but the relative weights applied to these measurements (e.g., the coefficients of discriminant functions) were derived from analysis of similar measurements made on other people. In the present context, predictions will be based entirely on the individual patient's own record of past measurements, provided this record contains at least the minimum number of observations required to make such a prediction. For example, when the record consists of only one earlier measurement of a given biochemical variable, we shall have to utilize within-person variances shown by a reference group in order to develop a statistical guideline for evaluating the second (current) measurement. In some cases, we shall also have to rely on the laboratory's quality control database to provide an estimate of the analytic component of the patient's within-person variability.

Repeated examinations imply that the patient is building up a record of results over time while remaining in steady state. The physician will be interpreting each new result in terms of its agreement or lack of agreement with the pattern of preceding results. When the latest observation is only the second in a series, there is obviously no "pattern" to go on, and interpretation relies on the simple numerical difference between the two results. At what point in time can a usable pattern be recognized, and how might agreement between the current result and the pattern of earlier results be tested statistically? These are questions to be explored in this chapter, primarily with respect to a single biochemical analyte. Since even a single analyte, when tested on more than one occasion, produces multiple results, the introduction of the time dimension creates its own kind of multivariate analysis. As we have seen in the previous chapter, dealing with several analytes on repeated occasions can lead to a complicated statistical problem. In theory, the solution may seem to be a straightforward extension of the method used for a single analyte. In practice, the brevity of most clinical series often makes it impossible to achieve a reliable description of a steady state pattern in multiple analytes. One exception, treated later in this chapter, is the case where, for each analyte, successive observations are mutually independent.*

Needless to say, the clinician or chemist reviewing serial laboratory data must expect to see some variability in the numbers even under acceptable steady state conditions. The causes of such variation are legion but may be broadly classified as either "physiological" or "analytical." The former class includes variations due to environmental, dietary, behavioral, and emotional effects, the latter variations in conditions under which specimens were collected, stored, or transported, as well as those during actual chemical analysis. Many such sources of variation can be controlled, thereby increasing sensitivity

---

*Univariate time series analysis may, of course, be applied to an index (e.g., a ratio) composed of two or more biochemical analytes.

to the real changes the clinician is looking for. For example, it is common in hospitals and ambulatory clinics, when dealing with patients in presumed steady state, to collect blood samples in the early morning after overnight fasting. Strenuous exercise should be avoided for 24 hours before the sample is taken (Statland et al., 1973). Restrictions on torniquet use and posture of the patient during blood collection have also been recommended [see Statland and Winkel (1977) for detailed discussions of practical procedures to control unwanted physiological and analytic effects]. Since interpretation of the test results will be based on observed change(s) rather than on a single individual value, any systematic bias in the chemical analysis is not important, provided the same instrumentation and biochemical method is used throughout the series of observations. Depending usually on the time interval between successive results, this may or may not be a problem. In many medical centers, however, different analytic systems are available to measure a given serum analyte, each with a different accuracy. In this situation, the transferability of results, or, more specifically, the numerical adjustments required to achieve comparable results, must be considered before an observed change can be properly interpreted.

Even after all precautions have been taken to reduce unwanted variability and assure comparability of serial measurements, the problem remains that the number of prior observations is often exceedingly small. They are not necessarily equispaced and may, in addition, be correlated with each other. In any case, clinical laboratory measurements are subject to random, uncontrolled biological and analytic factors. We consider the following four underlying parameters shaping an observed steady state pattern of a given analyte in the ith individual: (a) an underlying mean value μ_i around which the "true" concentrations (of which the measured values are estimates) fluctuate from time to time; (b) a correlation ρ_i between successive true concentrations; (c) a variance σ_{ei}^2 of small, but numerous, random biological effects; and (d) a variance σ_a^2 of similar analytic effects (usually called analytic imprecision).

We assume that, under steady state conditions, these parameters are constant over time. Mindful of the shortness of most clinical series, we incorporate them into a simple statistical structure, the first-order autoregressive model, written in two equations: one for the true concentration of the analyte in the ith individual at time t (say, m_{it}) and the other for its measured value x_{it}. Thus,

$$m_{it} = \mu_i + \rho_i(m_{i,t-1} - \mu_i) + e_{it} \tag{8.1}$$

$$x_{it} = m_{it} + a_t \tag{8.2}$$

where e_{it} and a_t are the net effects of uncontrolled biological and analytic factors, respectively, assumed to be normally distributed random variables with zero means and variances σ_{ei}^2 and σ_a^2. As indicated in the use of the subscript $(t - 1)$ in equation (8.1), we are also assuming at this point equispaced observations at some fixed time interval taken as a "unit" of time.

We will use these equations as our underlying model to describe ongoing steady state variation in an individual even when only two or three serial observations of the analyte are available (including the current one), too few to begin to identify a "pattern" of variation for that person. In fact, at least 10 to 15 repeated measurements are probably necessary to yield reliable estimates of the parameters defined above. Therefore, when later in this chapter we apply this model to individual series of fewer than ten observations, we shall reduce the model to two extreme cases which will, we hope, encompass the range of results available under the original form, equations (8.1) and (8.2).

At this point, having set forth some underlying concepts for dealing with individual series of clinical measurements, let us turn to consider the shortest possible series—two successive observations. Our problem is to develop an objective criterion for judging the observed change between initial and current measurements.

8.2 REFERENCE CHANGE VALUES

It appears from recent studies (Skendzel, 1978; Elion-Gerritzen, 1980; and Skendzel et al., 1985) that clinicians vary considerably in the amount of change between two successive measurements of a given analyte that they believe indicates the need for medical attention.

The smallest of these critical changes proposed by clinicians is often no greater than analytic error. For example, 45% of the doctors in both the Skendzel (1978) and Elion-Gerritzen (1980) studies would consider a change of 0.10 to 0.15 mmol/L in serum calcium (from an initial borderline normal value of 2.6 mmol/L) important enough to warrant medical follow-up. Assuming a coefficient of variation of 2% in calcium determination, the difference between two independent measurements at a level of 2.5 mmol/L would be subject to analytic imprecision of $\pm\sqrt{2}$ (0.05), or 0.07 mmol/L. When normal biological variability is included, a zero true difference could easily generate an observed difference of 0.1 to 0.15 mmol/L. On the other hand, in the most recent study (Skendzel et al., 1985), fully 50% of the physicians responding indicated that when evaluating results from asymptomatic patients undergoing routine annual physicals, they would not take any follow-up action unless the present calcium determination exceeded the previous year's by more than 0.4 mmol/L.

Working from the autoregressive time series model specified by equations (8.1) and (8.2), an objective criterion for change can be derived to replace these highly variable personal opinions. At the same time, as we shall see, considerable freedom of choice is retained. Since a single initial value cannot define a pattern for the individual patient, a reference population of similar patients will have to be considered at some point. To begin, let x_{it} denote the current (time t) measurement of analyte X in the ith patient, and $x_{i,t-1}$, the previous measurement at time $(t - 1)$, where the unit time interval may be a day, a week, a six-hour period, or whatever. Under the autoregressive model, the variance (standard deviation squared) of the difference $d_{i1} = x_{it} - x_{i,t-1}$ may be written

$$\text{var}(d_{i1}) = 2\sigma_i^2\{(1 - \rho_i) + \rho_i\sigma_a^2/\sigma_i^2\} \tag{8.3}$$

where σ_i^2, the variance of x_i over time, equals

$$\{\sigma_{ei}^2/(1 - \rho_i^2)\} + \sigma_a^2$$

In practice, the correlation ρ_i will be estimated from observations subject to measurement errors. The effect of such errors is to underestimate the true correlation by a factor of $\{1 - (\sigma_a^2/\sigma_i^2)\}$; that is, the expected value of the estimate $\hat{\rho}_i$ is equal to $\rho_i\{1 - (\sigma_a^2/\sigma_i^2)\}$. Substituting $\hat{\rho}_i\sigma_i^2/(\sigma_i^2 - \sigma_a^2)$ for ρ_i in equation (8.3), we obtain the much simpler result

$$\text{var}(d_{i1}) = 2\sigma_i^2(1 - \hat{\rho}_i) \tag{8.4}$$

so that knowledge of the analytic variance σ_a^2 is really unnecessary.

However, with only two observations available, there is no way of obtaining an estimate of the serial correlation, while σ_i^2 can only be estimated from the very difference whose randomness we are concerned about. Therefore, without additional information beyond the ith patient, the observed difference cannot be tested against its standard deviation. Suppose, however, that through past records of serial test results, we could obtain information on the distribution of within-person variances across a population of similar patients. The same data would provide individual estimates of the correlation ρ_i, which may be averaged to obtain a single estimate $\hat{\rho}$ for all patients. Selecting an appropriate value of σ_i^2, say $(\sigma_i^2)^*$ (for example, the 75th or 90th percentile), a "reference" standard deviation of d_{i1} could be calculated as $\{2(\sigma_i^2)^*(1 - \hat{\rho})\}^{1/2}$. Then, we define a "just significant difference" d_{i1}^* as equal to, say, twice this standard deviation. Since d_{i1}^* would be a "reference" change for all patients of a given type, we may omit the subscript i and write simply d_1^*, or $d_1^*(X)$ for analyte X. The details of obtaining $(\sigma_i^2)^*$ and $\hat{\rho}$ are described in Harris and Yasaka (1983).

An approach somewhat similar to this, called the "delta check," has been used in many clinical laboratories as a method of quality control (e.g., Nosanchuk and Gottmann, 1974; Ladenson, 1975; and Wheeler and Sheiner, 1977, 1981). The delta check is a critical difference between two successive test results, such that any observed difference exceeding this value signals a recheck of the laboratory's specimen identification and chemical analysis system for this patient and analyte. Sometimes the delta check value is chosen by reference to quality control data or by empirical "trial and error." In other laboratories, the value is selected by referral to the observed distribution of differences between two serial measurements of the analyte in patients recently at the hospital (Wheeler and Sheiner, 1981). For example, the 95th or 97.5th percentile of this distribution might be taken as the delta check value. The strength of this method lies in its simplicity. The laboratory must identify and accumulate paired values, then sort their differences, but no more complicated statistical procedures are involved. The distribution of differences already contains the effects of variations in within-person variances and of correlations between successive test results.

However, reported experience with delta check values obtained in this way has shown that many false alarms occur even when a reasonably high percentile difference is used. The reason for this derives from the very simplicity of the procedure. The overall distribution of differences will naturally reflect both small and large within-person variances and all in between. Small variances will tend to generate small differences between two successive values; large variances will generate large differences. As a result, the observed 95th percentile difference approximates the 95th percentile of a distribution of differences from a hypothetical population with a constant within-person variance equal to the average observed variance. However, if we actually generate a distribution of within-person variances from similar patients in steady state, we can specifically select $(\sigma_i^2)^*$ to be a high percentile of this distribution. Basing a reference change value on this choice of $(\sigma_i^2)^*$ is then like dealing with a distribution of differences from a hypothetical population of individuals all of whom possess large within-person variances. The delta check value from such a distribution of differences would be much larger than that from the real distribution, greatly reducing the probability of false alarms. Would it be too large, insensitive to real changes in the conditions of many patients?

With this question in mind, we present briefly some results of applying this reference change procedure to data from two sources: (a) a large health monitoring and maintenance program in Japan; and (b) a regional medical center in the United States. The former population consisted of healthy individuals pursuing their normal activities and tested every six months; the latter is represented by groups of inpatients from different services. Also included for comparison are delta check values obtained from the distribution of differences between adjacent test results in each patient.

A. Health Monitoring Program in Japan

Figure 8.1 shows the cumulative distribution of within-person variances in measurements of calcium, by sex (286 women, 412 men). Each variance is based on 15 to 18 semiannual health monitoring examinations of persons enrolled in the Perfect Liberty Health Control System with clinics in Osaka and Tokyo. The fairly linear plots on logarithmic probability paper indicate that these observed variances are approximately lognormally distributed. Since the means and variances of these two distributions were very similar, we combined the graphs into a single lognormal distribution, shown in Figure 8.2. However, this is now an estimated distribution of true within-person variances σ_i^2; the procedures used to convert the means and variances of observed variances to their estimated values for true variances are described in Harris and Yasaka (1983).

Now suppose, for example, that we select the 90th percentile of this distribution, 7.2×10^{-3} (mmol/L)^2. In these data, $\hat{\rho}$ was very close to zero, so that the corresponding reference change value would be $d_1^* = 2(2 \times 7.2 \times 10^{-3})^{1/2}$, or

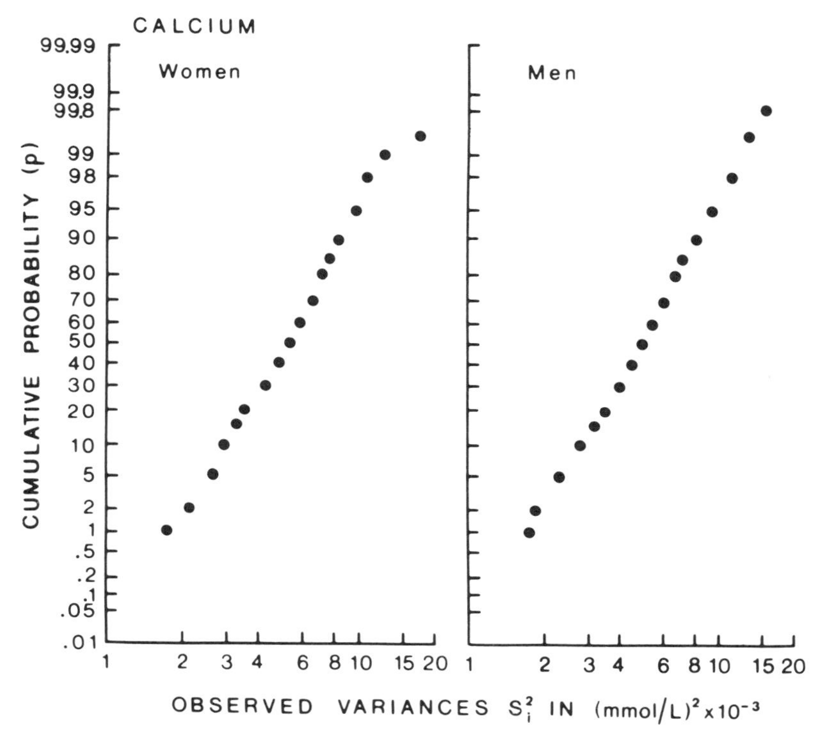

FIGURE 8.1 Cumulative probability distributions of within-person variances in semi-annual measurements of calcium, by sex (Harris and Yasaka, 1983).

0.24 mmol/L of calcium. Had we chosen the 75th percentile of σ_i^2 from Figure 8.2, the reference change would have been $d_1^* = 0.22$ mmol/L. Indeed, one may calculate a corresponding value of d_1^* for every percentile of σ_i^2, generating a distribution of possible reference changes for this analyte.

On the other hand, suppose we derived our reference change value directly from the distribution of differences between adjacent measurements. Using differences from non-overlapping pairs of consecutive observations (i.e., $x_2 - x_1$; $x_4 - x_3$, etc.), the 97.5th percentile of the distribution of differences was 0.20 mmol/L. This value corresponds to only the 35th percentile of σ_i^2 in this population. Even this value is

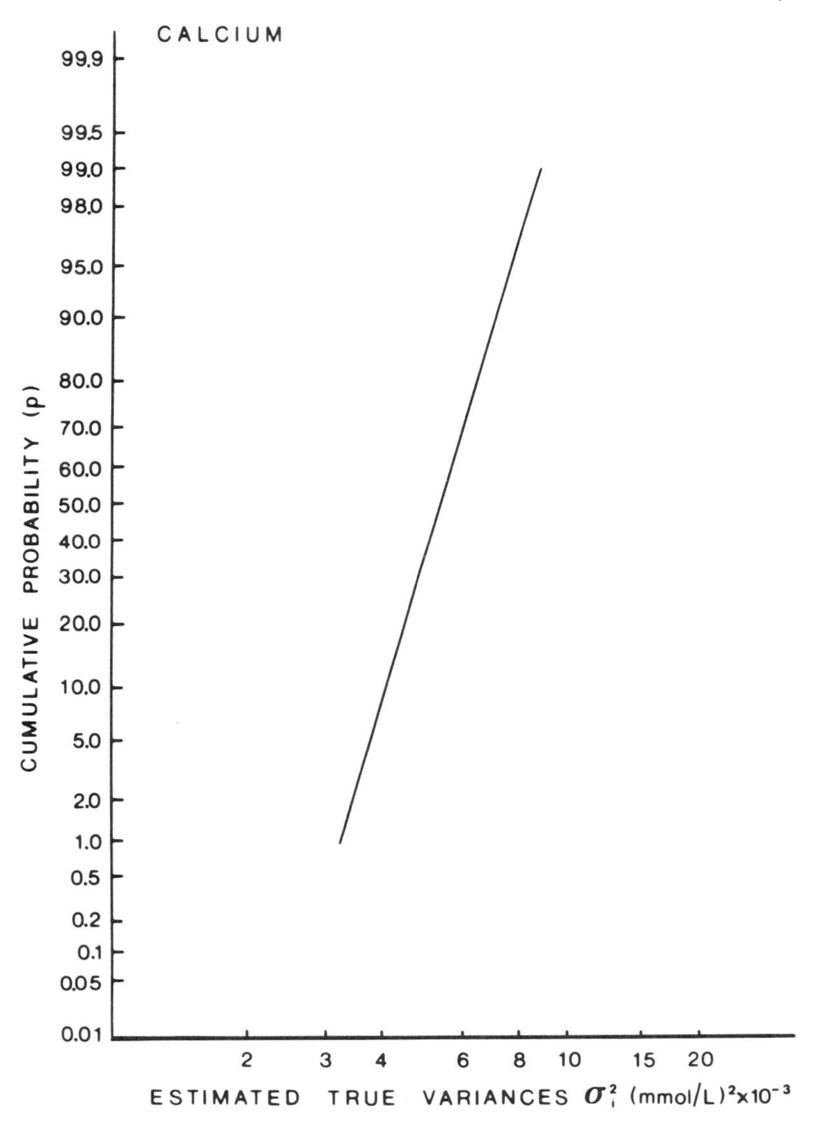

FIGURE 8.2 Estimated cumulative distribution of true within-person variances for calcium.

substantially greater than the "critical" differences chosen by almost half of the resident physicians queried in previously cited studies (Skendzel, 1978; and Elion-Gerritzen, 1980).

B. Regional Medical Center in the United States

In this study (Boyd and Harris, 1986), serial electrolytes, urea and creatinine measurements in patients from two different hospital services, a surgery ward, and a surgical intensive care unit, are being compared. The expectation is that patients recovering from plastic surgery will show much greater day-to-day stability in these analytes than will patients under intensive care. This would imply that a much smaller reference change would be appropriate for patients in the former class than in the latter. However, since our purpose here is simply to illustrate the idea of the reference change value, we will present data from one group only, the surgery patients. Figures 8.3(a) and (b) are lognormal probability plots (like Figures 8.1 and 8.2) of observed within-person variances and estimated true variances, respectively, of urea nitrogen (BUN) measurements in 51 patients. Each variance was computed from at least four successive results obtained at daily intervals. The distribution of observed variances appears skewed to the left (on log scale) due to some quite small values. However, the bulk of the variances seems approximately lognormal. The method used to estimate the mean and variance of this distribution (Healy, 1979) minimizes effects of discrepant extreme values by a trimming procedure. Figure 8.3(b), like Figure 8.2, assumes the underlying distribution of true variances to be lognormal.

Unlike the calcium data, the BUN series showed a high average correlation between consecutive daily values, $\hat{\rho} = 0.55$. Computation of the reference change value would then be based on the formula $2\{2(\sigma_i^2)^*(1 - \hat{\rho})\}^{1/2}$, given earlier. Setting $(\sigma_i^2)^*$ at the 90th percentile of the distribution in Figure 8.3(b), 34 $(\text{mg/dL})^2$, the corresponding reference change value $d_1^* = 2\{2 \times 34(1 - .55)\}^{1/2} = 11.1$ mg/dL. Using the 75th percentile of σ_i^2, 16.5 $(\text{mg/dL})^2$, $d_1^* = 7.7$ mg/dL. The

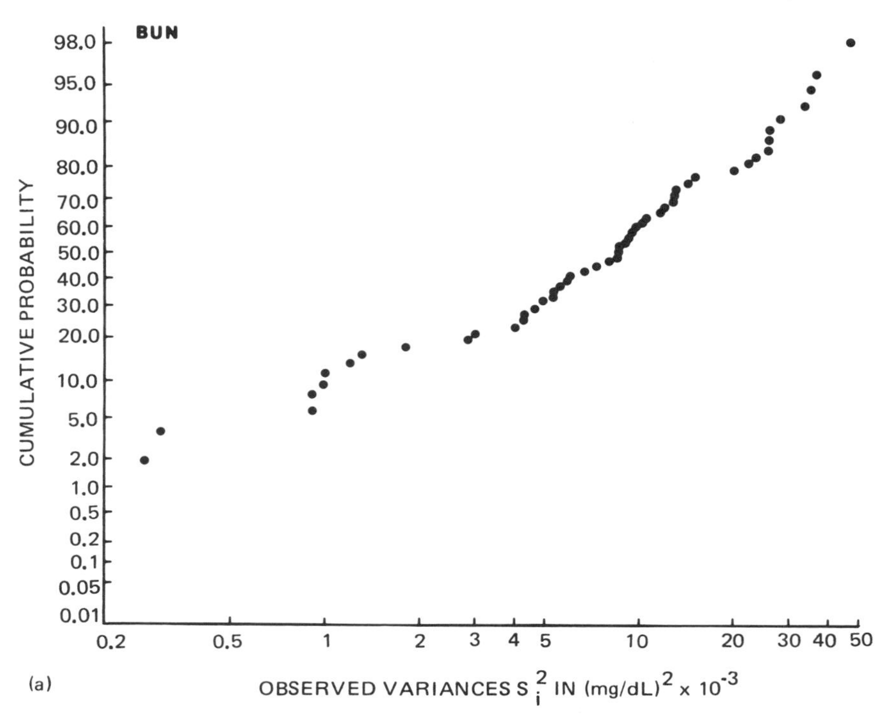

FIGURE 8.3 (a) Cumulative probability distribution of within-patient variances in daily measurements of urea nitrogen (BUN). (b) Estimated cumulative distribution of true within-patient variances for BUN (Harris and Yasaka, 1983).

97.5th percentile of differences from nonoverlapping pairs of consecutive observations was 5.0, corresponding to the 48th percentile of σ_i^2.

8.3 JUDGING A TREND IN THREE OBSERVATIONS

A "trend" in three successive measurements is simply an increasing or decreasing series of numerical results. This does not necessarily mean that the differences between first and second and second and third observations are equal, only that

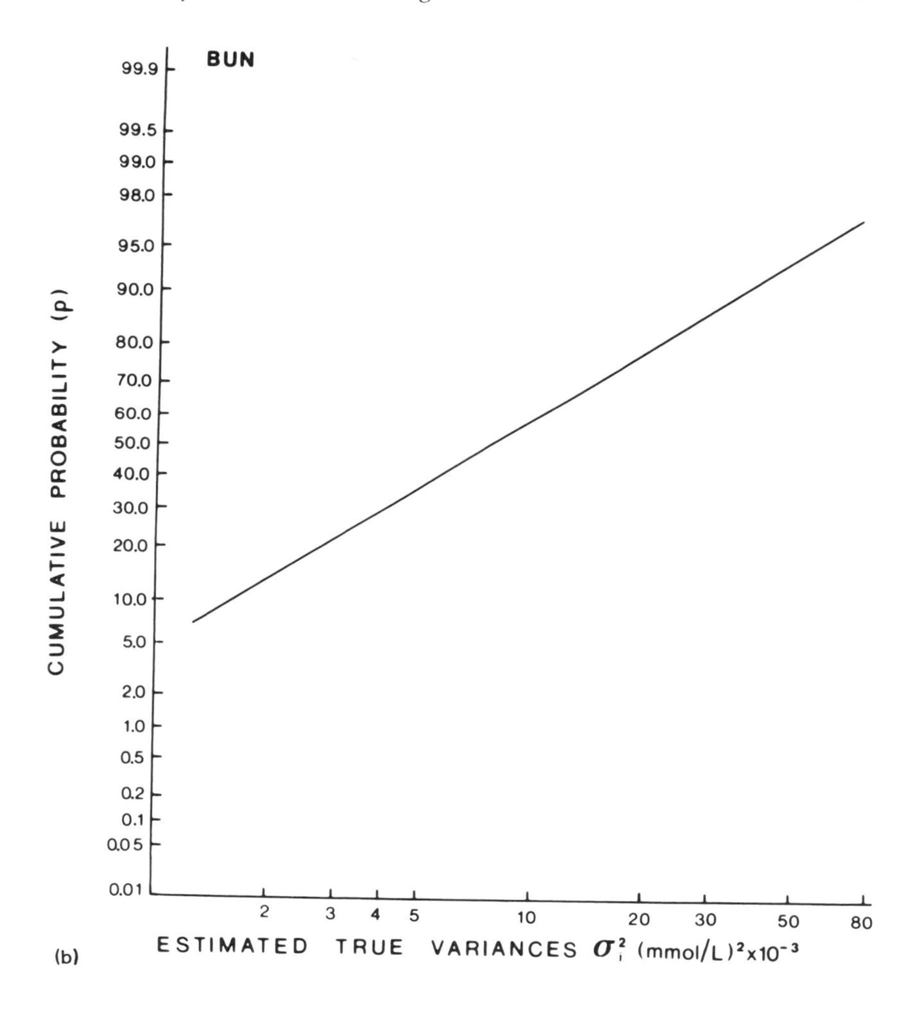

they are in the same direction. An extension of the method described above provides a reference criterion for judging the difference between first and third observations. A property of the first-order autoregressive model is that the serial correlation (when positive) declines exponentially as the time interval between measurements increases. Thus, if ρ_{12} denotes the correlation between two successive true concentrations of a given analyte, and ρ_{13} the correlation between two concentrations at twice the elapsed time interval, the model states that $\rho_{13} = \rho_{12}^2$. The correlation between two concentrations k time units apart is equal to ρ_{12}^k. If ρ_{12} is negative, the series of true values is oscillatory, and so is the correlation function.

It follows that, under the autoregressive model, the variance of the difference between first and third measurements, becomes

$$\mathrm{var}(x_{it} - x_{i,t-2}) = \mathrm{var}(d_{i2}) = 2\sigma_i^2\{(1 - \rho_i^2) + \rho_i^2\sigma_a^2/\sigma_i^2\} \qquad (8.5)$$

Correcting, as before, for the downward bias in the (average) estimate $\hat{\rho}$ obtained from observations subject to measurement errors, equation (8.5) becomes

$$\mathrm{var}(d_{i2}) = 2\sigma_i^2\{1 - \hat{\rho}^2\sigma_i^2/(\sigma_i^2 - \sigma_a^2)\} \qquad (8.6)$$

The estimated standard deviation obtained as the square root of the right-hand side of equation (8.6) will usually be greater than the standard deviation used to judge the change between first and second measurements [from equation (8.4)] but may be only slightly larger. This implies that a difference between the first two observations smaller than the reference change can, if repeated between second and third measurements, produce a significant overall trend. Of course, where $\hat{\rho}$ equals zero, as in the calcium data, the reference change value remains the same regardless of the time interval between the two observations.

8.4 WHEN THREE OR MORE PRECEDING OBSERVATIONS ON THE SAME PATIENT IN STEADY STATE ARE AVAILABLE

With at least three serial observations available while the patient is in steady state, a barely sufficient basis exists to define a pattern against which succeeding measurements may be judged without bringing in additional information from a population of other patients. We are chiefly concerned with the question of whether a current deviation from the preceding pattern is large enough to merit further medical attention.

We will outline a statistical approach to answering this question, but, of course, the medical importance of a numerical deviation can only be decided by the pathologist or clinician. Before this, the clinical chemist or other member of the laboratory staff will have checked to be sure that the observed deviation did not arise from some purely technical circumstance in the laboratory, such as misidentification of the specimen or a change in analytic method. Thus, the immediate benefit of a statistical criterion, like all reference guidelines, should be to alert the laboratory staff to a possible problem.

Using the autoregressive model, we should like to forecast the likely range of values of the current observation x_t if, in fact, the steady state described by the preceding observations has continued through time t. If x_t lies outside this range, we conclude that a statistically significant change has occurred in the patient's condition, at least as far as analyte X is concerned. Unfortunately, even the simple autoregressive model described by equations (8.1) and (8.2) involves too many unknown parameters for practical use as a forecasting device when only a small number of serial observations are available. We can partly resolve the difficulty by considering two extreme forms of the model, obtained by setting ρ equal to zero or to one.

Each of these extreme cases will produce a forecast range; one will usually lie entirely within the other. The upper and lower bounds of the wider range should encompass the next (current) observation even if the actual generating process is better described by an autoregressive model in which ρ lies between zero and one.

A. $\rho = 0$: Independent Observations

When $\rho = 0$, all serial observations are mutually independent. The model reduces to the single equation,

$$x_t = \mu + e_t + a_t \tag{8.7}$$

omitting the subscript i because it is now understood that we are restricting ourselves to data from a single individual. Under this model, called by statisticians the "white noise" model, we cannot estimate the variance components σ_e^2 and σ_a^2 separately but only their sum. Given $t - 1$ preceding observations, their variance s_{t-1}^2 around the observed mean $\bar{x}_{t-1}$ estimates this combined variance. The mean itself, with estimated variance $s_{t-1}^2/(t - 1)$, is our best (minimum variance) estimate of the homeostatic setpoint, as well as the best predictor of the observation at time t, assuming no change in the process. However, to calculate a forecast range we should also include the variability of individual measurements, estimated by s_{t-1}^2. Therefore, under the white noise model, the forecast range becomes

$$\bar{x}_{t-1} \pm \tau_{\alpha,t-2}\, s_{t-1} \{t/(t - 1)\}^{1/2} \tag{8.8}$$

where $\tau_{\alpha,t-2}$ denotes "Student's t" at significance level α and degrees of freedom $t - 2$.* When t is as small as 4 or 5 (i.e., only three or four serial observations preceding the current one), the value of τ at the usual two-sided significance levels ($\alpha = 0.05$ or 0.01) is so large that the resulting forecast ranges would be too wide for practical use. However, if we increase α (the "error of false rejection of the null hypothesis") to, say, 0.1 for a two-sided test, then $\tau = 3$ would be appropriate for $t = 4$ and $\tau = 2.4$ for $t = 5$. If medical importance is attached to a deviation of the analyte in only one direction, these combinations of τ and t would be proper for $\alpha = 0.05$ and a one-sided forecast.

B. $\rho = 1$: Nonstationary "Random Walk" Model

When ρ is set equal to one in equation (8.1), the underlying mean μ disappears, and we are left with the statement that the true concentration at time t is equal to the true

---

*The classical notation for Student's t percentage points, $t(\alpha;\upsilon)$, has been deliberately changed to avoid the confusion with the time factor t.

concentration at the previous sampling time except for a random biological disturbance. The absence of a homeostatic "setpoint" throughout the entire period of observation places this extreme case in the category of "nonstationary" time series models. To indicate this, we should in fact replace the symbol e_t, which represents a random deviation from a stationary setpoint, by another symbol, say Δ_t, denoting a short-term shift from the preceding concentration value, which was itself shifted from a still earlier value. Thus, each of the concentrations m_1, $m_2, \ldots, m_t$ is assumed to be entirely determined by its value in the immediate past plus a change due to transient random circumstances. There is no "centripetal" force pulling the concentration at any time to some underlying long-term position. This can result in apparent drifts over a few sampling times which are, in fact, entirely random, do not reflect a change from "normal" to pathological conditions and could very well reverse direction in the near future. Such a pattern of results has been called, in modern statistical texts, a "random walk," or, in earlier works, the "drunkard's path." When serial observations show a nondirectional pattern, the random walk model will generate a forecast range wider than that under the homeostatic model. When observations show a trend, however, the random walk presumes continuation of the trend, even though it is a random event, and indicates this by a narrower forecast range.

There may seem little reason to expect random walk behavior in a series of biochemical test results from an individual, but the model becomes more appropriate with increasing correlation between successive values. Let us think of a random physiological deviation as the effect of a temporary disturbance to an otherwise homeostatic system. Then the correlation between two successive concentration values depends on the time it takes for this effect to wear off, compared to the elapsed time between measurements. The higher the ratio of these two times, the larger the correlation between two successive concentrations. The "decay time" of a disturbance varies among analytes. Some, like cholesterol, react slowly to disturbances (dietary changes, for example) but also recover slowly. Such analytes tend to show higher serial correlations than others, like serum electrolytes, which react and recover much more quickly because close adherence to homeostasis in electrolyte balance is vital to the organism. In general, a shorter time interval between measurements will produce higher correlations than a longer interval, but again this depends on the analyte.

As discussed above, we shall write the random walk model in the form

$$m_t = m_{t-1} + \Delta_t \tag{8.9}$$

$$x_t = m_t + a_t \tag{8.10}$$

where Δ_t, the shift in true values, is assumed to be normally distributed with mean zero and variance σ_Δ^2 (Harris, 1981). Under this model, the best estimate of the concentration at time t, say $\hat{m}_t$, will be obtained by weighting the observation x_t by some fraction $w_t \leq 1$ and earlier observations x_{t-k} ($k = 1, 2, 3, \ldots$) by exponentially declining weights w_t^{k+1}. This method, called "exponential averaging," was widely used as a forecasting procedure long before it was shown (Muth, 1960) to be optimal for the random walk model. It is still a popular smoothing device for any series of correlated observations, whether from a stationary or nonstationary process. The estimating formula may be condensed to the recursive form

$$\hat{m}_t = w_t x_{t-1} + (1 - w_t)\hat{m}_{t-1} \tag{8.11}$$

The estimate $\hat{m}_t$ also becomes our forecast for the next observation x_{t+1}. To determine w_t, we recall that an optimal weighted average is obtained when each weight is the reciprocal of the variance of the term to which it is applied, divided by the sum of the reciprocals so that the weights sum to unity. This implies that w_t should equal

$$\frac{\text{var}(\hat{m}_{t-1})}{\text{var}(x_t) + \text{var}(\hat{m}_{t-1})}$$

Now, x_t as an estimator of m_t will have variance σ_a^2, whereas $\hat{m}_{t-1}$ as an estimator of m_t will have variance equal to its variance as an estimator of m_{t-1} plus σ_Δ^2, the variance of the shift from m_{t-1} to m_t. By going back to $\hat{m}_1 = x_1$, then $\hat{m}_2 = w_2x_2 + (1 - w_2)x_1$, and proceeding step by step, we find that the variance of $\hat{m}_{t-1}$ as an estimator of m_t equals $w_{t-1}\sigma_a^2 + \sigma_\Delta^2$ (Stewart, 1970). Hence,

$$\begin{aligned} w_t &= \frac{w_{t-1}\sigma_a^2 + \sigma_\Delta^2}{w_{t-1}\sigma_a^2 + \sigma_\Delta^2 + \sigma_a^2} \\ &= \frac{w_{t-1} + c}{w_{t-1} + c + 1} \end{aligned} \tag{8.12}$$

where $c = \sigma_\Delta^2/\sigma_a^2$ and $w_1 = 1$. For practical application to short series, we have to assume σ_a^2 known and estimate σ_Δ^2 and c sequentially from the observations (see example below).

The forecast range for an observation at time t under this model must, as before, include not only the variance of the predicted value $\hat{m}_{t-1}$ but also the variance of individual observations about their true mean m_t. Since this variance is σ_a^2, the $100(1 - \alpha)\%$ forecast range becomes

$$\hat{m}_t \pm \tau_{\alpha,t-2}\, \sigma_a\, (w_{t-1} + \hat{c}_{t-1} + 1)^{1/2} \tag{8.13}$$

The primary characteristic of these calculations, regardless of which model is being used, is their sequential nature. If a new observation lies within its forecasted range, we accept it as a continuation of the preceding pattern and use it to update our knowledge of the current state of the system. Updating variances is a key operation because the variances of observations represent the variances of disturbances to the system. In the "white noise" model, we noted that the variance of the observations up to and including time $(t - 1)$ estimates the sum of analytic and biological variances required to obtain the forecast range at time t. The random walk model is nonstationary in the original observations, but successive differences $d_1 = x_t - x_{t-1}$ are stationary with mean zero and variance equal to $\sigma_\Delta^2 + 2\sigma_a^2$. Assuming σ_a^2 known, we may estimate σ_Δ^2 by subtracting $2\sigma_a^2$ from the variance of observed d_1 values (called the variance of "first" differences). In general, differences between observations k time units apart are stationary under the random walk model with mean zero and variance $k\sigma_\Delta^2 + 2\sigma_a^2$, a result that is helpful in adapting the model to a series with missing observations (see next section).

To simplify sequential calculation of observed means and variances, we can take advantage of two results from elementary statistics:

1. The mean:

$$\begin{aligned}\bar{x}_t &= \left\{ \left(\sum_{j=1}^{t-1} x_j\right) + x_t/t \right\} \\ &= \{(t-1)\bar{x}_{t-1} + x_t/t\}\end{aligned} \tag{8.14}$$

2. Given two groups: n_1 observations with mean $\bar{x}_1$ and variance s_1^2, and n_2 observations with mean $\bar{x}_2$ and variance s_2^2, the variance of all $n_1 + n_2$ observations together is given by

$$s^2 = \frac{1}{n_1 + n_2 - 1} \left\{(n_1 - 1)s_1^2 + (n_2 - 1)s_2^2 + \frac{n_1 n_2}{n_1 + n_2}(\bar{x}_1 - \bar{x}_2)^2\right\} \tag{8.15}$$

Now suppose that the first group contains $(t - 1)$ observations with mean $\bar{x}_{t-1}$ and variance s_{t-1}^2, while the second group contains only one, the t-th observation x_t. Then $\bar{x}_2 = x_t$, $s_2^2 = 0$, and the pooled variance becomes

$$s_t^2 = \frac{1}{t - 1} [(t - 2)s_{t-1}^2 + \{(t - 1)/t\}(\bar{x}_{t-1} - x_t)^2] \qquad (8.16)$$

Therefore, to update the mean and variance with each new observation, it is unnecessary to maintain all previous observations but only the preceding mean and variance, starting with $\bar{x}_1 = x_1$ and $s_1^2 = 0$. Of course, the same formula can be used when dealing with differences, as in updating the estimate of σ_Δ^2 (or $c = \sigma_\Delta^2/\sigma_a^2$) in the random walk model.

To illustrate the use of these procedures, we have selected cholesterol series from two persons who were undergoing periodic health monitoring examinations at 6 to 12-month intervals during the early 1970's. [These and other data have been presented in Harris (1976) where they are discussed in greater detail.] To keep the calculations as simple as possible, we shall ignore the variability in time intervals between successive observations; the adjustment for missing observations is taken up in the next section. The data consist of five observations in each series, listed in Table 8.1. One can see immediately that B showed much greater within-person variation than A, although neither series appears to be trending up or down. Initial estimates are derived from the first three observations in each series. Each succeeding observation (assuming it falls within its forecast range) is then used to update these estimates and calculate a forecast range for the next observation. Successive results for $t = 3$, 4, and 5 are given below the data.

The calculations for equation (8.7), the autoregressive model with $\rho = 0$, are relatively simple. The predicted value for the observation at time t is equal to the mean of the preceding $(t - 1)$ observations. Thus, in series A for $t = 4$, the predicted value is 192.33. The corresponding standard error of prediction, using equation (8.8), is the standard deviation of the preceding $(t - 1)$ observations, multiplied by $\{t/(t - 1)\}^{1/2}$. For $t = 4$, $S.E. = (3.06)(4/3)^{1/2} = 3.53$, leading to a forecast range of $192.33 \pm 2.92 \times 3.53 = 182.0 - 202.6$,

TABLE 8.1 Applying Equations (8.8; Homeostatic Model) and (8.11–8.13; Random Walk Model) to Two Individual Cholesterol Series

Series A					
t	Obs. (x_t) (mg/dL)	d_{i1} ($x_t - x_{t-1}$)	Mean	S.D.	w
1	193	—	193	0	1
2	195	2	194	1.41	0.5
3	189	−6	192.33	3.06	0.333
4	204	15	195.25	6.34	0.843
5	200	−4	196.2	5.89	0.816

	Equation (8.8)		Equations (8.11–8.13)	
t	Predicted value	S.E.	Predicted value	S.E.
4	192.33	3.53	192.3	4.62
5	195.25	7.09	202.2	10.48
6	196.2	6.45	200.4	9.31

Forecast ranges (predicted value $\pm\ \tau_{\alpha,\,t-2}$ S.E.)[a]			
t	τ	Equation (8.8)	Equation (8.13)
4	2.92	182.0 to 202.6	178.8 to 205.8
5	2.35	178.6 to 211.9	177.6 to 226.8
6	2.13	182.5 to 209.9	180.6 to 220.2

Series B					
t	x_t	d_{i1}	Mean	S.D.	w
1	207	—	207	0	1
2	160	−47	183.5	33.23	0.993
3	182	22	183.0	23.52	0.993
4	208	26	189.25	22.91	0.991
5	192	−16	189.8	19.88	0.987

TABLE 8.1 *(continued)*

t	Equation (8.8) Predicted value	Equation (8.8) S.E.	Equations (8.11–8.13) Predicted value	Equations (8.11–8.13) S.E.
4	183.0	27.16	181.9	48.79
5	189.25	25.62	207.8	41.04
6	189.8	21.78	192.2	34.49

Forecast ranges (predicted value $\pm\ \tau_{\alpha,\ t-2}$ S.E.)[a]

t	τ	Equation (8.8)	Equation (8.13)
4	2.92	103.7 to 262.3	39.4 to 324.4
5	2.35	129.0 to 249.5	111.4 to 304.2
6	2.13	143.4 to 236.2	118.7 to 265.7

[a] $\tau_{\alpha,\ t\ -\ 2}$ = Student's "t" at level of significance $100(1\ -\ \alpha)\%$ and $(t\ -\ 2)$ degrees of freedom. For these very short series, we have chosen $\alpha = 0.1$ (two-sided test), or $\alpha = 0.05$ (one-sided test).

as given in the table. Note that the observed value at $t = 4$, 204 mg/dL lies just outside this range. However, this small deviation from the previous pattern of results would not be considered clinically important. Including this observation with the earlier results increases within-person variability and produces a wider forecast range for the observation at $t = 5$.

For the random walk model [equations (8.9) and (8.10)], the calculations are a little more complicated, requiring the successive differences shown in the third column of Table 8.1 and their running variances (not shown). Updated values of $\hat{c} = \{\text{var}(d_{1i})/\sigma_a^2\} - 2$ are then computed. The analytic error σ_a was set at ± 4 mg/dL (CV of 2%) based on past experience in this laboratory with the measurement procedure for cholesterol. Weights w (column 6) are calculated sequentially from equation (8.12), followed by the predicted value [equation(8.11)] and forecast range (8.13) for each new observation.

Because of the very large within-person variation relative to analytic variance, $\hat{c}$-values are high, leading to weights almost equal to unity. The predicted value at a given sampling time is then practically the same as the preceding observed value but with a rather large error of estimate (*S.E.*) and wide forecast range. Note that these ranges include the correspondingranges from equation (8.7) and encompass all observed results.

For series *B*, both models produce extremely unlikely lower limits, but the upper limits under equation (8.7) are quite realistic at all times and at $t = 6$ under the random walk model. Thus, a jump in the next (sixth) cholesterol measurement in this patient to above 240 mg/dL should be considered medically significant, certainly if above 265. In series *A*, on the other hand, a sixth observation above 220 would indicate an increase worth attention even though such a value lies well within the conventional "normal range" based on a cross section of healthy persons.

The random walk model is relatively insensitive to errors in the choice of analytic standard error, σ_a. For example, if the laboratory had actually determined these cholesterol values with a CV of 4% rather than 2%, the upper limits of the forecast ranges under this model in series *A* would have changed by less than 5%. In series *B*, with its much greater biological variation, the changes would have been less than 0.3%.

8.5 MISSING OBSERVATIONS

Most series of biochemical or physiological observations in a given patient are planned to follow a periodic schedule, e.g., every eight hours, every morning, every six months. In practice, of course, the intervals will only be approximately equal, but the discrepancies should be small relative to the scheduled time span between observations. It often happens, however, that an observation is not taken at or near the planned time, so that a gap of two or three times the scheduled interval appears at various points in the series. In some series, such gaps are "built in," for example, when tests are done at the same time each weekday, or every four hours during the day-time. In the white noise model ($\rho = 0$), gaps can be ignored.* In the random walk model, gaps may be taken into account fairly easily, as follows.

Suppose that observations have been more or less equally spaced up to a certain time $t - n$, but that the next observation was not obtained until n time units later at time t. The predicted value for this observation would be $\hat{m}_{t-n}$, but what forecast range should be put around this prediction? Now, as we saw earlier, the variance of m_{t-1} as an estimator of the true value at the next scheduled sampling time is given by $w_{t-1}\sigma_a^2 + \sigma_\Delta^2$, where the latter term represents the variance of biological fluctuations within the time interval. When n time intervals have elapsed since the last observation, the variance of $\hat{m}_{t-n}$ as an estimator of m_t will be $w_{t-n}\sigma_a^2 + n\sigma_\Delta^2$. Adding in the analytic variance associated with the observation x_t, the appropriate forecast range becomes

$$\hat{m}_{t-n} \pm \tau_{\alpha,t-n-1}\, \sigma_a\, (w_{t-n} + n\hat{c}_{t-n} + 1)^{1/2} \tag{8.17}$$

Assuming that the new observation fell within this forecast range, how would we incorporate it with preceding data to obtain a new estimate of m_t? As before, this would be a weighted average, $\hat{m}_t = w_t x_t + (1 - w_t)\hat{m}_{t-n}$, where the weight

$$w_t = \frac{\text{var}(\hat{m}_{t-n})}{\text{var}(\hat{m}_{t-n}) + \text{var}(x_t)} \qquad \text{as an estimator of } m_t$$

$$= \frac{w_{t-n}\sigma_a^2 + n\sigma_\Delta^2}{w_{t-n}\sigma_a^2 + n\hat{\sigma}_\Delta^2 + \sigma_a^2} = \frac{w_{t-n} + n\hat{c}_t}{w_{t-n} + n\hat{c}_t + 1}$$

The estimate $\hat{m}_t$ also becomes the predicted value of x_{t+1}, hedged by a $100(1 - \alpha)\%$ forecast range given by

---

*That is, only actual observations are taken into account when updating time t in equations (8.7) and (8.8).

$$\hat{m}_t \pm \tau_{\alpha,t-n}\, \sigma_a\, (w_t + \hat{c}_t + 1)^{1/2} \tag{8.18}$$

These equations presume that the estimate $\hat{c}$ is available from preceding data. The question arises how to utilize measurements separated by gaps (integral multiples of a fixed time interval) to update prior estimates of c. As noted earlier, with observations at a fixed interval we would estimate c from the variance of first differences: $\hat{c} = \{\text{var}(d_1)/\sigma_a^2\} - 2$. Each new observation would generate recomputation of var(d_1) and an updated estimate of c. When the data series includes gaps, only a portion of the values can contribute to the calculation of var(d_1). For example, observations isolated between two gaps cannot be included at all. They may contribute to the variances of differences between observations separated by more than one time interval, but such variances will be less stable than var(d_1). It does not seem worthwhile to try to develop a weighted average estimate of c including estimates based on variances other than var(d_1). When the time interval between observations is irregular with no evidence of periodicity, no direct estimate of c is possible. An iterative maximum likelihood procedure has been described by Jones (1983) for multivariate time series considered below.

Clearly the forecasting process can get quite tedious if missing observations occur frequently with gaps of varying length. Existing computer programs deal with this situation by replacing missing datapoints with some pseudovalue (e.g., 9999), alerting the program to use the appropriate formulas.

8.6 EXTENSION TO THE MULTIVARIATE TIME SERIES

As mentioned earlier, time series analysis of even one biochemical quantity is already multivariate because it deals with multiple observations, any pair of which may be strongly or weakly correlated. We may expect therefore that a unified statistical treatment of more than one concurrent series would be a very complex task because we would have to account for serial correlations within each variable as well as cross-correlations among variables. The situation becomes relatively simple in one important case, multivariate "white noise," because this model assumes that all serial correlations are zero. The statistical methodology for sequential analysis of such data has been described by Harris et al. (1982). Since the variances of the different analytes over time have to be estimated as well as the covariances between concurrent pairs of values, we recommend an initial base of no fewer than five serial observation vectors. This would probably be considered much too sparse a database by most time series analysts, and indeed it is for any multivariate model more complicated than white noise. However, in many health monitoring programs, where clinical laboratory data may be collected only every six months or at even longer intervals, five serial observation vectors represent a considerable passage of time. This may also be true in patient monitoring where laboratory tests are run more frequently but the medical problem is more acute so that early detection of a significant deviation becomes especially important.

Under white noise models, unequally spaced sampling times do not create a problem, assuming that even the longest interval between observations is short compared to the time span for long-term changes (e.g., aging effects). Therefore, we need to consider only the number of sampling times, denoting this by n. The predicted value of the vector of observations at the n-th sampling time is the vector of mean values through the preceding $(n - 1)$ times. Call this $\bar{\mathbf{x}}_{n-1}$. Let $\mathbf{S}_{n-1}$ represent the variance–covariance matrix of differences between observed and predicted vectors through these $(n - 1)$ times. The "distance" between the vector at the nth sampling time and its predicted value is given by

$$D_n^2 = (\mathbf{x}_n - \bar{\mathbf{x}}_{n-1})^T \mathbf{S}_{n-1}^{-1} (\mathbf{x}_n - \bar{\mathbf{x}}_{n-1}) \tag{8.19}$$

where $\mathbf{x}_n$ is the nth column vector of observations and $\mathbf{S}_{n-1}^{-1}$ is the inverse of the matrix $\mathbf{S}_{n-1}$. The null hypothesis states that the deviation of the nth observed vector from its forecast is simply a random sample from a k-variable Gaussian distribution, k being the number of biochemical analytes included. The test statistic used is

$$F_{n,k} = \{(n - 1)/n\} (n - k - 1) D_n^2/k(n - 2) \qquad (8.20)$$

which is distributed under the null hypothesis in an F-distribution with k and $(n - k - 1)$ degrees of freedom (Chew, 1966). If $F_{n,k}$ exceeds the tabled value of F at the chosen level of significance (say, 0.05), we conclude that the multivariate vector of current observations represents a statistically significant departure from the pattern of results seen up to that time. Note that when $k = 1$—the univariate case—the square root of $F_{n,1}$ reduces to Student's t statistic (called τ in this chapter) that we used in that case to calculate a forecast range.

8.7 MULTIVARIATE ANALYSIS WITH SERIALLY CORRELATED OBSERVATIONS

Application of the general autoregressive model or the nonstationary random walk model to a multivariate time series is, in our opinion, not yet practical for clinical laboratory data, except perhaps in research studies. The reasons are two-fold. First, the minimum length of time series required for estimation of parameters is too long for routine use; at least twenty serial vectors are needed. Second, computer programs currently available are not only quite complicated and costly to operate, but more important, they are not sequential in nature. Instead, estimates are derived from an initial database and then applied to forecast a series of future values. The programs may be modified to run in sequential mode, but the cost of repeated reestimation of parameters could be very high because of the nonlinear iterative estimation procedures required.

The major statistical theory and methods in this area have been published by Jones (1966, 1985) in two valuable papers. The first of these deals with the multivariate random walk model applied to equispaced observations. Jones's estimation procedure does not require that analytical variances be known. The second paper extends this work to the general first-order autoregressive model, with white noise and random walk models as special cases. The theory accommodates irregularly spaced observation vectors and includes a chi-square test to judge whether the general autoregressive model fits the data significantly better than either of the special cases. Iterative maximum likelihood estimating procedures are used and computer programs are available, as noted above.

8.8 SPECIFICITY/SENSITIVITY OF MULTIVARIATE VERSUS UNIVARIATE TIME SERIES MODELS AND THE PROBLEM OF REPEATED SIGNIFICANCE TESTS

In Chapter 3, we noted that cross-sectional multivariate reference regions were likely to include vectors in which one or more test results lay outside their respective univariate ranges. In other words, multivariate regions tend to be more "conservative" than multiple univariate ranges, implying that the sporadic false positive result for one analyte will probably be "washed out" when combined with results from other analytes and referred to a multivariate reference region. As we mentioned, this is usually a good thing since we know that as the number of tests increases, so too does the probability of at least one false positive result. On the other hand, when a laboratory test is ordered to help confirm or rule out a particular diagnosis, it hardly makes sense to include other tests unrelated to the diagnosis and then refer the observed vector to a multivariate reference range. This can only obscure a real signal by mixing it with "noise." We discussed this in Chapter 3 but call attention to it again here because multivariate and univariate time series analyses relate to each other in this respect exactly as do cross-sectional reference regions (e.g., see Harris et al., 1982).

There is an additional aspect to this problem in the case of serial results. As we noted above, such data represent a multivariate situation even when only one analyte is involved. As more and more observations are made over time, each tested against its forecast range, the probability of finding a result outside its range by chance alone increases. Now, a one-step-ahead forecast range at any time is independent of earlier one-step-ahead ranges (Box and Jenkins, 1976), so this increase of probability can be computed as if from a set of independent analytes, each being tested against its own reference range. It would seem that the practical answer to this problem is not to widen each successive forecast range, but rather to require out-of-range results in at least two successive test results, or else to demand corroborative evidence from other sources, before concluding that the patient's state has been significantly altered. The situation is comparable to that in laboratory quality control (e.g., Westgard et al., 1981).

In recent work on the application of equation (8.7) (the autoregressive model with $\rho = 0$) to post-operative monitoring, Winkel et al. (1982) recognized the problem posed by repeated significance tests and suggested a solution involving two threshold (upper) limits at each sampling time. Their study concerned women operated on for breast cancer from whom monthly blood and urine samples had been collected and analyzed in an effort to detect any recurrence of the disease as soon as possible. Various enzymes and other constituents were measured, but only the tumor marker CEA (cancerembryonic antigen) showed any changes related to recurrence.

The authors postulated a fixed series of ten samples and proposed setting two thresholds, one relatively high so that a single "out-of-control" value would not be falsely taken as an indication of recurrence, another much lower to trap series in which an actual recurrence had generated at least two consecutive or three nonconsecutive high values. The probability of either type of event occurring while the patient remained in a nonrecurrent state was set at 0.05 or 0.01 as desired. The two threshold levels were calculated from simultaneous binomial probability equations. Although fixing an a priori limit on the number of serial samples to be examined does not jibe with sequential analysis of results as they occur, these equations could be solved for various lengths of series and some reasonable compromise reached on threshold levels.

Both the sensitivity and specificity of this modified application of equation (8.7) were estimated. The total number of women included in this study was not large, but the authors' findings were supported by a computer-simulation that made use of an exponential model for the rate of growth of the tumor since tumor size was thought to influence the level of CEA in the blood. All in all, this study represents pioneering work in a quite new area of application of statistical theory to laboratory medicine.

8.9 A TWO-TIERED UNIVARIATE RANDOM WALK MODEL

Before closing this chapter, it may be worthwhile to mention briefly an elaboration of the univariate random walk model that has appeared in the recent literature in connection with the analysis of serial clinical laboratory data. This model was originally introduced in a purely statistical context by Harrison and Stevens (1976) and consists of three equations:

$$\begin{aligned} x_t &= m_t + a_t \\ m_t &= m_{t-1} + \Delta_t + \beta_t \\ \beta_t &= \beta_{t-1} + \delta_t \end{aligned} \tag{8.21}$$

Comparison with the equations of the random walk model shows that a random slope term β_t has been introduced, which, like the true value m_t, follows a random walk over time. A third variance σ_δ^2 enters in addition to σ_a^2 and σ_Δ^2. Smith and West (1983) have used this model to monitor serum creatinine as an indicator of renal function in patients who have received kidney transplants. They distinguish among four candidates for the state of the system at any given sampling time: (1) steady state; (2) change in level; (3) change in slope; and

(4) outlier. For example, a substantial slope change will suddenly increase σ_δ^2 and thereby sharply increase the probability corresponding to this state relative to those for the other states. These state probabilities, recomputed sequentially, are the primary output for clinical attention. Their computed values depend in part on arbitrary (but experience-based) numerical settings for the relative magnitudes of the variance terms under different possible states. The sequential estimating formulas for the probabilities are derived from basic principles of Bayesian estimation applied to Gaussian-distributed random variables. These formulas appear quite forbidding to those who are not serious students of Bayesian statistical theory. The methodology for estimating the current true value of the system, and the standard error of that estimate, is a special case of "Kalman filter" theory described in the previously-cited paper by Harrison and Stevens (1976).

A simpler application of the same model has been reported by Harris (1981). The variable was also serum creatinine as an indicator of kidney dysfunction but in a patient with systemic lupus erythematosus. Renal complications in this disease usually proceed much more slowly than in patients receiving transplants. The emphasis was on sequential estimation of the parameters m_t and β_t, then testing of these estimates against their standard errors in traditional fashion. Initially unstable estimates of the variances σ_Δ^2 and σ_δ^2 (σ_a^2 assumed known) were obtained from the variances of second and third differences. However, these appeared to settle down quickly as further observations were enlisted. The Kalman filter equations were used to estimate m_t, β_t, and their standard errors. Results were compared with those from the random walk model without a slope term.

8.10 CONCLUDING REMARKS

More and more work is being reported on statistical analysis and interpretation of longitudinal clinical laboratory data, especially as familiarity with sequential Bayesian estimation techniques grows among practicing statisticians (see, for example, the expository article on Kalman filtering by Meinhold and Singpurwalla, 1983). The size and complexity of the required computer programs may impede more widespread application of these methods to multivariate observation vectors, but more important will be the cost of rerunning the program package as each new observation vector appears. The advantages of a large, efficient central facility to which many remote workstations (terminals with video displays and printers) may be connected will be apparent here, but the cost may still be too high for routine use in the near future. What is perhaps most exciting in these pioneering days of the subject is that there now exist methods for sequential analysis and assessment of the stream of clinical data collected during patient management. Further advances in theory and technique will undoubtedly appears. The routine use of stochastic (i.e., nondeterministic) time series methods in hospital laboratories will focus on single analytes before venturing to multivariate batteries of tests, and much will depend on good display systems. Comprehensive computer-based cumulative reporting systems are essential, as is the ability to develop selected databases from past laboratory records so that results appropriate to different kinds of patients can be obtained. Given these important technical assets, problems in the interpretation of serial test results can now be addressed with sound statistical methods tailored to meet real clinical needs.

REFERENCES

Box, G. E. P., and Jenkins, G. M. (1976). *Time Series Analysis, Forecasting and Control,* Second Edition. Holden-Day, San Francisco.

Boyd, J. C., and Harris, E. K. (1986). Utility of reference change values for the monitoring of inpatient laboratory data. In Optimal Use of the Clinical Laboratory, O. Zinder (Ed.). Karger, Basel.

Chew, V. (1966). Confidence, prediction and tolerance regions for the multivariate normal distribution. *J. Amer. Stat. Assoc. 61*, 605–617.

Elion-Gerritzen, W. E. (1980). Requirements for analytical performance in clinical chemistry. *Amer. J. Clin. Pathol. 73*, 183–195.

Harris, E. K. (1981). Further applications of time series analysis to short series of biochemical measurements. In *Reference Values in Laboratory Medicine: The Current State of the Art*, R. Grasbeck and T. Alstrom (Eds.). John Wiley, New York, pp. 167–176.

Harris, E. K. (1976). Some theory of reference values. II. Comparison of some statistical models of intraindividual variation in blood constituents. *Clin. Chem. 22*, 1343–1350.

Harris, E. K., and Yasaka, T. (1983). On the calculation of a "reference change" for comparing two consecutive measurements. *Clin. Chem. 29*, 25–30.

Harris, E. K., Yasaka, T., Horton, M. R., and Shakarji, G. (1982). Comparing multivariate and univariate subject-specific reference regions for blood constituents in healthy persons. *Clin. Chem. 28*, 422–426.

Harrison, P. J., and Stevens, C. F. (1976). Bayesian forecasting (with discussion). *J. Royal Stat. Soc., Series B, 38*, 205–247.

Jones, R. H. (1966). Exponential smoothing for multivariate time series. *J. Royal Stat. Soc., Series B, 28*, 241–251.

Jones, R. H. (1985). Fitting multivariate models to unequally spaced data. In *Proceedings of the ONR Symposium on Time Series Analysis of Irregularly Spaced Data, February 10–13, 1983*, E. Parzen (Ed.). Springer-Verlag, New York.

Ladenson, J. (1975). Patients as their own controls: Use of the computer to identify "laboratory error." *Clin. Chem. 21*, 1648–1653.

Meinhold, R. J. and Singpurwalla, N. D. (1983). Understanding the Kalman filter. *Amer. Statistician 37*, 123–127.

Muth, J. F. (1960). Optimal properties of exponentially weighted forecasts. *J. Amer. Stat. Assoc. 55*, 297–306.

Nosanchuk, J. S., and Gottmann, A. W. (1974). CUMS and delta checks. *Amer. J. Clin. Pathol. 62*, 707–712.

Skendzel, L. P. (1978). How physicians use laboratory tests. *JAMA 239*, 1077–1080.

Skendzel, L. P., Barnett, R. N., and Platt, R. (1985). Medically useful criteria for analytic performance of laboratory tests. *Amer. J. Clin. Pathol. 83*, 200–205.

Smith, A. F. M., and West, M. (1983). Monitoring renal transplants: An application of the multiprocess Kalman filter. *Biometrics 39*, 867–878.

Statland, B. E., and Winkel, P. (1977). Effects of non-analytical factors on the intra-individual variation of analytes in the blood of healthy subjects. Consideration of preparation of the subject and time of venipuncture. *CRC Crit. Rev. Clin. Labor. Science 8*, 105–144.

Statland, B. E., Winkel, P., and Bokelund, H. (1973). Factors contributing to intra-individual variation of serum constituents. II. Effects of exercise and diet on variation of serum constituents in healthy subjects. *Clin. Chem. 19*, 1380–1383.

Stewart, K. B. (1970). A new weighted average. *Technometrics 12*, 147–157.

Westgard, J. O., Barry, P. L., Hunt, M. R., and Groth, T. (1981). A multi-rule Shewhart chart for quality control in clinical chemistry. *Clin. Chem. 27*, 493–501.

Wheeler, L. A., and Sheiner, L. B. (1981). A clinical evaluation of various delta check methods. *Clin. Chem. 27*, 5–9.

Wheeler, L. A., and Sheiner, L. B. (1977). Delta check tables for the Technicon SMA 6 continuous-flow analyzer. *Clin. Chem. 23*, 216–219.

Winkel, P., Bentzon, M. W., Statland, B. E., Mouridsen, H., and Sheike, O. (1982). Predicting recurrence in patients with breast cancer from cumulative laboratory results: A new technique for the application of time series analysis. *Clin. Chem. 28*, 2057–2067.

A Last Word

The statistical theory and methods described in this book may seem at times to involve a strong dose of mathematical machinery, much of it probably unfamiliar to the clinical chemist or physician. The reason lies primarily in the multivariate nature of the data to be analyzed. Once we require the statistical analysis to deal in a unified, coordinated way with multiple variables, then, for the sake of generality, we must assume that the variables are not independent of each other in the probability sense. That is, their joint probability distribution is not simply the product of their respective univariate distributions but is a more complex form involving new parameters, which describe the varying degrees of nonindependence between variables.

Forced by the essential nature of the problem to become involved in rather complicated mathematical formulations, the statistical analyst of clinical laboratory data must find some way to bridge the inevitable communications gap between himself (or herself) and his audience, the chemist/clinician. Like many others, we have usually done this by "boiling down" the analysis ultimately to a single number, a probability—specifically, a posterior probability or predictive value. In some cases, we end up with a predictive range bounded by two numbers. Time series analysis of successive measurements allows plotting these predictive probabilities or intervals sequentially, thus increasing their attractiveness and usefulness in patient management. Further opportunities for graphical display, presenting the univariate results as well as multivariate indices, should also be considered in reporting laboratory data.

We believe predictive probabilities and ranges represent not only objective summaries of the data but, more importantly, powerful guidelines to help the attending physician reach optimal decisions given the facts at hand. Another whole system of clinical data interpretation is to be found in computerized "knowledge bases" supplemented by rules for evaluating data and formulating medical decisions. Although in any particular field of application the knowledge base may be supplied by specialists in that field, the concepts underlying the storage of this information and development of appropriate decision rules are part of the general science of artificial intelligence (Rich, 1983). The purpose is to simulate and, in practice, improve upon the ability of the trained human brain to comprehend a variety of new data, to weigh, at least roughly, the importance of each bit of information, and to evaluate the whole against stored knowledge and experience. The result may be to seek further data or to consider a set of appropriate decisions, each with a calculated probability of being correct. The entire process, outlined too briefly here, comprises an "expert" system for a given area of application. Two well-known examples are CADUCEUS (Pople, 1982), formerly known as INTERNIST, developed for internal medicine by Miller et al. (1982), and MYCIN, a program that attempts to recommend appropriate therapies for patients with bacterial infections (Shortliffe, 1976).

Clearly, the potential scope of such systems is wider than any of the statistical analyses discussed in this book. Indeed, perhaps they attempt too much, inviting a protective reaction from the physician. On the other hand, statistical techniques for interpretation of clinical data have their own possible drawbacks. See, for instance, Spiegelhalter and Knill-Jones (1984) for a comprehensive review of this problem. Discriminant function analysis based on data from one group of patients may not be transferable without change to another patient population or another set of measurement devices. Its linear structure may be too restrictive, although this can often be modified and is, in any case, a good first approximation. Time series modeling applied to repeated measurements (either biochemical or physiological function tests) to detect early deviations from the patient's own norm, avoids most criticisms addressed to other statistical methods. However, as we have pointed out, multivariate time series analysis with serial correlation among successive observation vectors is not only complicated mathematically but, in sequential mode, makes heavy demands on computer time, even with large computers. It is probably not reliable for any multivariate series with fewer than 20 time points of observation.

Finally, a full understanding of discriminant analysis, or even time series analysis based on the simple univariate models mentioned here, requires more extensive training in statistical theory than most physicians or clinical chemists today can claim or may wish to have. In the end, of course, the results are simple guidelines, which the clinician, who has a richer store of knowledge about the individual patient and similar patients, may ignore, act upon, or modify as he or she thinks best.

A key characteristic of the medically oriented expert system is its interactive, sequential mode of application, allowing both computer system and clinical user to adapt to each other's approach and store of knowledge relative to the patient. It would seem reasonable, therefore, that statistical analyses intended to guide medical decisions be included within such expert systems. It is not entirely clear, however, that the rule-development processes inherent in expert systems (at least, as we understand them) can logically incorporate these statistical analyses, especially when the latter are directed toward serial observations. Until the feasability and usefulness of combining these developments have been confirmed, we think it probably better to continue to gain practical experience with each approach separately. We emphasize especially the importance of sequential analysis of patient data, yielding predictive probabilities or ranges with every new observation vector. The brevity of most clinical data series and the dynamic nature of the patient's response to illness or treatment each limit the applicability of multivariate theory in this area. To encourage use of that portion of theory that is appropriate to clinical data requires flexible, interactive programming that keeps the user in control. This, we feel, should be our continuing goal.

REFERENCES

Miller, R. A., Pople, H. E. Jr., and Myers, J. D. (1982): INTERNIST-1, an experimental computer-based diagnostic consultant for general internal medicine. *N. Eng. J. Med. 307,* 468–476.

Pople, H. E. (1982): Heuristic methods for imposing structure on ill structured problems: The structuring of medical diagnosis. In *Artificial Intelligence in Medicine,* (P. Szolovits, Ed.). Westview Press, Colorado, pp. 119–185.

Rich, E. (1983). *Artificial Intelligence.* McGraw-Hill, New York.

Shortliffe, E. H. (1976): *Computer-based Medical Consultations: MYCIN.* Elsevier, New York.

Spiegelhalter, D. J. and Knill-Jones, R. P. (1984): Statistical and knowledge-based approaches to clinical decision-support systems, with an application to gastroenterology (with Discussion). *J. Roy. Stat. Soc. A147,* 35–77.

APPENDIX

COMPUTER PROGRAMS

A. INTRODUCTION

This appendix describes two important computer programs that permit the application of some of the methods described in this book. They have been included mainly because, to our knowledge, they cannot be found in general statistical packages like SAS, BMDP, GLIM, or SPSS.

The first program, LOGDIS, performs multiple group logistic discrimination, a multivariate statistical method referred to several times in this book, particularly in Chapter 5. The program also allows the user to calculate likelihood ratio functions, described in Chapter 4. To illustrate application of the methods, the program was run on the liver enzyme data appended to Chapter 5.

The second program, TIMSER, applies statistical methods described in Chapter 8 for the analysis of equidistant serial laboratory data. It handles both homeostatic (white noise) and random walk models for univariate time series. As an example, the program was applied to the cholesterol data presented in Chapter 8. A modified program to deal with series containing gaps (see Section 8.5 of Chapter 8) is available on request from the authors.

Programs related to the other multivariate methods described in this book can sometimes be found in existing statistical packages. For instance, the program P7M of BMDP performs classical multivariate normal discriminant analysis (see Chapter 5). If programs for specific tasks discussed here are not available in these packages, the relevant formulas and equations are easily programmable using, for example, the SAS procedures. The current availability of statistical packages and procedures on personal computers considerably widens the potential use of multivariate methods for clinical laboratory data. References to statistical packages include the following:

1. Baker, R. J., and Nelder, J. A. (1978). *General Linear Interactive Modelling (GLIM)*, Release 3. Numerical Algorithm Group (NAG), Oxford.

2. Dixon, W. J., and Brown, M. C. (1979). *Biomedical Computer Programs,* P-Series (*BMDP*). University of California Press, Berkeley.
3. Nie, N. H., Hull, C. H., Jenkins, J. G., Steinbrenner, K., and Bent, D. H. (1975). *Statistical Package for the Social Sciences* (*SPSS*). McGraw-Hill, New York.
4. *SAS User's Guide: Statistical Analysis System* (1979). SAS Institute, Inc., Cary, North Carolina.

B. LOGDIS: A MULTIPLE GROUP LOGISTIC DISCRIMINATION PROGRAM

Description of Program

Object

The program performs multiple group logistic discrimination. In discriminant analysis, the problem is to find a rule for allocating a multivariate observation $\mathbf{x}^T = (x_1, \ldots, x_k)$ into one of g groups, say $H_1, \ldots, H_g$. It is assumed that a sample of observations is available from each group.

Logistic Model

The logistic approach to discrimination offers the advantage of being applicable to a large family of multivariate distributions, involving discrete or continuous variables or a mixture of both. It is based on the assumption that the posterior probabilities are a generalized logistic function of linear combinations of the variables, i.e.

$$\mathrm{pr}(H_s|\mathbf{x}) = \frac{a_{0s} + \mathbf{a}_s^T\mathbf{x}}{\sum_{t=1}^{g} \exp(a_{0t} + \mathbf{a}_t^T\mathbf{x})} \qquad s = 1, \ldots, g \qquad (1)$$

where $\mathbf{a}_s^T = (a_{1s}, \ldots, a_{ks})$, and by convention $a_{0g} = 0$ and $\mathbf{a}_g = \mathbf{0}$. As seen from equation (1), in the g-group situation, there are $g - 1$ discriminant functions (or scores) $l_s(\mathbf{x}) = a_{0s} + \mathbf{a}_s^T\mathbf{x}$. There is only one in the classical two-group problem.

Estimation

Under model (1), there are $(k + 1) \times (g - 1)$ parameters to estimate. The method used is the maximum likelihood (ML) estimation method. The likelihood function is maximized using a classical Newton-Raphson iterative procedure.

References

A description of model (1) and ML estimation of its parameters can be found in the following references:

1. Day, N. E., and Kerridge, D. F. (1967). A general maximum likelihood discriminant. *Biometrics 23,* 313–323.
2. Anderson, J. A. (1972). Separate sample logistic discrimination. *Biometrika 59,* 19–35.
3. Albert, A., and Anderson, J. A. (1984). On the existence of maximum likelihood estimates in logistic regression models. *Biometrika 71,* 1–10.

Program Characteristics

The program is conversational and is written in Fortran IV for PDP-11 and DEC-10/20 computers. With only minor changes, it can be readily implemented on any other computer system (e.g., VAX, IBM, HP).

Structure

The program is structured on the following elements:

a. a main program LOGDIS, interacting with the user and gathering the data needed for the logistic discrimination.

This program also prints information about the database and lists the original data, scores, and posterior probabilities, depending on the user's requests;

b. a subroutine LOGMLE, which actually performs the maximum likelihood estimation of the coefficients of the discriminant functions. All results of the Newton-Raphson iterative procedure are printed by the routine;

c. a set of utility subroutines LOGPRO, LOGI01, LOGI02, LOGI03, LOGI04, LOGI05, LOGI06, LOGI07, LOGI08, DFLOAT, INDICE, PRCHI2, PRGAMA, and DGAMA, called by LOGDIS and LOGMLE. The subroutines LOGI02, LOGI03, LOGI08, and PRGAMA originally appeared as algorithms in various issues of the *Journal of the Royal Statistical Society,* Series C (Applied Statistics). They are reproduced here with kind permission of the Royal Statistical Society. Complete references are given in the listing of LOGDIS immediately following this description.

Database Requirements

LOGDIS requires the database to be structured as follows. For each record in the file, there is (a) a patient identification, read in A-format (max A6); (b) a group number, read in I-format (max I3); (c) the values of the variables $x_1, \ldots, x_k$, read in F-format (max F10).

Dialogue

In LOGDIS, the user must provide the following elements:

1. FILE: the name of the file containing the dataset (20A1)
2. KG: the total number of groups (I2)
3. GNAME: the names of the groups, one per line (20A4)
4. NV: the total number of variables (I2)*

---

*Later in the program, only a subset (NVAR) of these variables may be used in the discriminant analysis (see point 10 below).

5. XNAME: the names of the variables, one per line (20A4)

6. FMT: the format of the data to be read in (10A8). It should consist of the following elements: (a) patient identification, in A-format, (b) patient group number, in I-format, and (c) the values of the variables, in F-format.

7. NG,(IG(I),I = 1,NG): the number of codes and the values of these codes (5I3) that will be used for group H_1; then repeat for group H_2, and so on. This way, it is possible to use different codes to create the groups. For example, if in the file the group codes are 1,2,3,4, and 5, we may like to compare $H_1 = (1,2,4)$ with $H_2 = (3,5)$. So for group H_1, we enter 003001002004, and for group H_2, we enter 002003005.

8. IDATA: a binary variable (I1) such that,
—if IDATA = 0, the program will print the original observations, the posterior probabilities $\text{pr}(H_s|\mathbf{x})$, $s = 1, \ldots, g$, and the scores $l_s(\mathbf{x})$, $s = 1, \ldots, g - 1$ for all observations.
—if IDATA = 1, no print.

9. ITYP: a binary variable (I1) indicating the type of sampling scheme,
—if ITYP = 0, we assume that there is mixture sampling, that is, all observations are drawn from the MIXTURE $H = (H_1, \ldots, H_g)$. If n_s denotes the number of observations from H_s, then the prior probability of H_s is $p_s = n_s/n$, where $n = n_1 + \cdots + n_g$.
—if ITYP = 1, we assume that the samples have been drawn SEPARATELY from each group H_s. This implies that the priors must be supplied by the user and sum up to 1. (PRIOR(I),I = 1, KG): priors are read in F-format, one per line.*

---

*If ITYP = 1, the results are affected in two ways: (i) the estimated independent terms a_{0s}, $(s = 1, \ldots, g - 1)$ and their asymptotic variance-covariances are subject to minor adjustments, and (ii) the posterior probabilities change with different priors. See also the section on likelihood ratio functions for additional information.

10. NVAR,(LIST(I),I = 1,NVAR): The number of variables used in the discriminant analysis (NVAR), chosen among the NV variables read in, and the list of their codes (LIST(I),I = 1,NVAR) in format (20I2). Thus, if 15 variables have been read in and discriminant analysis is to be performed on the 4 variables, 1,7,9, and 14, then enter 0401070914.
11. ISDX: a binary variable (I1) such that:
—if ISDX = 0, the statistical analysis is made on the original matrix of observations.
—if ISDX = 1, the program computes the mean and standard deviation of all variables across the entire dataset and standardizes all variables to zero mean and unit variance.*

Exit from the Program

The program loops on the elements 10–11 described above. To exit the program, type 0 (zero) in reply to question 10. So if NVAR = 0, the program stops. All results can then be retrieved from the file FOR06.DAT.

Divergence

The program is able to detect complete and quasicomplete separation in the dataset, situations in which the iterative process diverges, because ML estimates do not exist. When a warning message appears with ISDX = 0, rerun the program with ISDX = 1 and see whether there is genuine quasicomplete separation or whether the ML estimates exist and are finite. Complete and quasicomplete separation in logistic discriminant analysis are described in reference (3).

---

*Setting ISDX = 1 often improves convergence and enables the detection of quasicomplete separation in the data. When ISDX = 1, the program provides the coefficients not only for the transformed variables but also for the variables in original units.

Units Used

Four input and output channels, which can be combined or modified by the user, are used in the program: channel 1, disk file containing the dataset; channel 4, the screen for printing messages and questions; channel 5, the screen or a disk file used for inputting elements 1 to 11; and channel 6, the screen or a disk file containing the results of the analysis.

Dimensions

Initially the program is written for a maximum of 5 groups, 10 variables, and a matrix of observations of 600 elements. Instructions are given in the program listing for changing these dimensions to any size, depending on the computer capacity and resources available.

Example

The program LOGDIS was run on the hepatitis dataset listed in Appendix I of Chapter 5. Only the first three groups (acute viral hepatitis, persistent chronic hepatitis, aggressive chronic hepatitis) were envisaged, and the variables were AST, ALT, and GLDH. The input data below are the responses (on channel 5) to the elements 1–11 described in the "dialogue" section above.

Element No.	Data to be input
1	HEPATIC.DAT
2	03
3	ACUTE VIRAL HEPATITIS
	PERSISTENT CHRONIC HEPATITIS
	AGGRESSIVE CHRONIC HEPATITIS
4	03
5	AST
	ALT
	GLDH

Element No.	Data to be input
6	(A6,I4,3F10.0)
7	001001
	001002
	001003
8	0
9	0
10	03010203
11	0
10	00 (to stop the program)

The results of the run of LOGDIS on these data can be seen on the output listing below.

The Likelihood Ratio Function

The program LOGDIS can also be used to determine the likelihood ratio function for interpreting clinical laboratory data. Given a k-dimensional vector $\mathbf{x}^T = (x_1, \ldots, x_k)$, a disease D and its complementary state $\overline{D}$, it is assumed that the likelihood ratio, $L(\mathbf{x}) = \mathrm{pr}(\mathbf{x}|D)/\mathrm{pr}(\mathbf{x}|\overline{D})$, has the exponential form

$$L(\mathbf{x}) = \exp(a_0 + a_1 x_1 + \cdots + a_k x_k) \tag{2}$$

where $(a_0, a_1, \ldots, a_k)$ is a set of unknown parameters to be estimated from samples of observations from D and $\overline{D}$.

Program Input

The responses given to elements 1–11 of LOGDIS are similar to those used for multiple group discriminant analysis, but the following instructions should be carefully observed.

1. FILE: identical
2. KG: always set equal to 02

3. GNAME: give first name of group D, then the name of group $\overline{D}$
4. NV: identical
5. XNAME: identical
6. FMT: identical
7. NG,(IG(I),I = 1,NG): give first codes for group D, then for group $\overline{D}$
8. IDATA: identical
9. ITYP: must be set equal to 1 and followed on the next two lines by priors also equal to 1.0
10. NVAR,(LIST(I),I = 1,NVAR): identical
11. ISDX: identical, usually set equal to 0.

Example

As an illustration, the program LOGDIS was used to determine the likelihood ratio function between acute viral hepatitis (group D, $n = 57$) and (persistent + aggressive) chronic hepatitis (group $\overline{D}$, $n = 84$) on the basis of ALT only. The likelihood ratio function obtained is (see final matrix of coefficient B on listing)

$$L(\text{ALT}) = \exp(-1.953 + 0.0062\ \text{ALT})$$

and the standard errors of the coefficients were 0.3364 and 0.0011, respectively. The final classification matrix (with cutoff point $L = 1$) is also given in the program output. Likewise, the likelihood ratio function based on AST and ALT is given by the equation

$$L(\text{AST},\text{ALT}) = \exp(-2.272 - 0.0142\ \text{AST} + 0.0156\ \text{ALT})$$

The input data to obtain these two equations in one run of the computer program are given below:

Element No.	Data to be input
1	HEPATIC.DAT
2	02
3	ACUTE VIRAL HEPATITIS (GROUP D)
	CHRONIC HEPATITIS (GROUP DBAR)
4	03
5	AST
	ALT
	GLDH
6	(A6,I4,3F10.0)
7	001001
	002002003
8	1
9	1
	1.0
	1.0
10	0102
11	0
10	020102
11	0
10	00 (To stop the program)

Listing of Program and Subroutines (Fortran)

```
C                     P R O G R A M    L O G D I S
C
C***********************************************************************
C
C     PROGRAM FOR PERFORMING MULTIPLE GROUP LOGISTIC DISCRIMINATION
C
C***********************************************************************
C
C     VERSION: January 1986
C
C     REFERENCES: (1) Anderson, JA (1972). Separate sample logistic
C                     discrimination. Biometrika 59, 19-35
C                 (2) Albert, A and Anderson, JA (1984). On the existence
C                     of maximum likelihood estimates in logistic
C                     regression models. Biometrika 71, 1-10
C
C     ****************************************************************
C
C     THIS CONVERSATIONAL PROGRAM IS WRITTEN IN FORTRAN IV FOR DEC-10
C     AND PDP-11 COMPUTER SYSTEMS. WITH ONLY MINOR CHANGES, IT CAN BE
C     IMPLEMENTED ON ANY OTHER MACHINE (VAX, IBM, HP, ETC.)
C
C     UNITS: 1=DSK: INPUT FILE CONTAINING THE DATASET
C            4=TTY: TERMINAL MESSAGES
C            5=TTY: OR DSK: INSTRUCTION INPUT FILE
C            6=DSK: OUTPUT FILE CONTAINING THE RESULTS
C
C     ROUTINES CALLED: LOGIO1, LOGIO6, LOGIO7, LOGIO8, LOGMLE, LOGPRO
C
C     FOR EACH SUBJECT THE PROGRAM READS "NV" VARIABLES (IN VECTOR Y).
C     HOWEVER, LATER ON THE PROGRAM CAN BE RUN ON ANY SUBSET OF THESE
C     VARIABLES (IN VECTOR X). THUS WHEN COMPARING LOGISTIC DISCRIMINANT
C     FUNCTIONS OBTAINED WITH DIFFERENT SUBSETS OF VARIABLES, THE NUMBER
C     OF SUBJECTS INVOLVED IS ALWAYS THE SAME. BY CONVENTION, MISSING
C     VALUES SHOULD BE CODED -5.0 AND WILL LEAD TO THE REJECTION OF THE
C     COMPLETE MULTIVARIATE OBSERVATION.
C
C     DIMENSIONS: IF NV=NO. VARIABLES, KG=NO. GROUPS, NOBS=TOTAL NO.
C                 OF OBSERVATIONS, NV1=NV+1, KG1=KG-1,
C                 THEN WE HAVE THE FOLLOWING DIMENSIONS:
C
C     DATA(NV),LIST(NV),LISTX(NV),XBAR(NV),SD(NV),XNAME(20,NV),KSI(KG)
C     B(NV1*KG1),PSI(KG),PRIOR(KG),GNAME(20,KG),LISTG(KG),ERR(KG,KG),
C     N(KG),NPAT(NOBS),X(NOBS*NV1),Y(NOBS*NV1),LISTC(NV1),BC(NV1*KG1),
C     XB(NV*KG),STD(NV*KG),NT(KG),TWT(KG)
C
C     NOTE: IN THIS VERSION NV=10, KG=5, NOBS*NV1=600.
C
C***********************************************************************
C
```

```
      IMPLICIT REAL*8(A-H,O-Z)
      REAL*8 KSI(5)
      DIMENSION FMT(10),DATA(10),X(600),B(44),LIST(10),PSI(5)
      DIMENSION PRIOR(5),XBAR(10),SD(10),LISTC(11),BC(44)
      DIMENSION XB(50),STD(50),NT(5),TWT(5)
      REAL*4 XNAME(20,10),GNAME(20,5),NUMRO,NPAT(200),Y(600)
      INTEGER ERR(5,5),CITIT,N(5),IG(5),CYCLE,LISTG(5),LISTX(10)
      LOGICAL*1 FILE(20),DAY(9),HOUR(8)
      COMMON/RESULT/ERR,ISEP,IQSEP,IWARN,IERROR,CITIT,RLL1
C
C       DETERMINE DATE AND TIME OF RUN
C
      CALL DATE(DAY)
      CALL TIME(HOUR)
C
C       READ DATASET FILE NAME (FILE).
C
      WRITE(4,700)
      READ(5,500)FILE
      CALL ASSIGN(1,FILE)
C
C       READ PROBLEM SPECIFICATIONS: NUMBER OF GROUPS (KG) AND
C       NAMES (GNAME), TOTAL NUMBER OF VARIABLES (NV) AND NAMES
C       (XNAME), FORMAT OF INPUT DATA IN FILE (FMT).
C
      WRITE(4,701)
      READ(5,501)KG
      WRITE(4,702)
      DO 1 I=1,KG
1     READ(5,502)(GNAME(J,I),J=1,20)
      WRITE(4,703)
      READ(5,501)NV
      WRITE(4,704)
      DO 2 I=1,NV
      LISTX(I)=I
2     READ(5,502)(XNAME(J,I),J=1,20)
      WRITE(4,705)
      READ(5,503)FMT
      NV1=NV+1
      L=0
      K=0
      KG1=KG-1
      CYCLE=1
C
C       LOOP ON GROUPS (1 TO KG), READ DATA FROM FILE, CHECK IF NO
C       MISSING OBSERVATIONS, ALLOCATE TO CORRECT GROUP.
C
      DO 7 JK=1,KG
      LISTG(JK)=JK
      N(JK)=0
      REWIND1
      WRITE(4,706)JK
      READ(5,504)NG,(IG(I),I=1,NG)
```

```
3       READ(1,FMT,END=7)NUMRO,NGROUP,(DATA(J),J=1,NV)
C
C         CHECK WHETHER VECTOR (DATA) IS COMPLETE. IF NOT, REJECT.
C
        CALL LOGIO7(DATA,NV,ICHECK)
        IF(ICHECK.GT.0)GOTO3
C
C         VECTOR COMPLETE. CHECK TO WHICH GROUP IT BELONGS.
C
        DO 4 J=1,NG
        IF(NGROUP.EQ.IG(J))GOTO5
4       CONTINUE
        GOTO3
C
C         VECTOR ACCEPTED, UPDATE GROUP SAMPLE SIZE AND SAVE INTO
C         EXTENDED "1" VECTOR Y. ("1" NEEDED FOR INDEPENDENT TERM).
C
5       N(JK)=N(JK)+1
        K=K+1
        Y(K)=1.DO
        DO 6 J=1,NV
        K=K+1
6       Y(K)=DATA(J)
        L=L+1
        NPAT(L)=NUMRO
        GOTO3
7       CONTINUE
C
C         WARNING MESSAGE ON SCREEN
C
        IDIM=L*NV1
        WRITE(4,713)IDIM
C
C         ALL OBSERVATIONS HAVE BEEN PROCESSED.
C         ANSWER FURTHER QUESTIONS ABOUT THE OUTPUT OF RESULTS.
C
C         1. PRINT DATA MATRIX AND POSTERIOR PROBABILITIES (Y OR N).
C         2. SAMPLING TYPE: MIXTURE (ITYP=0), SEPARATE (ITYP=1).
C         3. STANDARDIZE DATA MATRIX (ISDX=1) OR NOT (ISDX=0).
C
        NOBS=0
        DO 8 I=1,KG
8       NOBS=NOBS+N(I)
        WRITE(4,707)
        READ(5,505)IDATA
        WRITE(4,708)
        READ(5,505)ITYP
        IF(ITYP.EQ.0)GOTO10
C
C         ITYP=1, SEPARATE SAMPLING SCHEME. READ PRIORS.
C         THE PRIORS SHOULD SUM UP TO ONE. THE CHECK FOR
C         A SUM EQUAL TO 2 IS ARTIFICIAL AND USED FOR THE
```

```
C          COMPUTATION OF A LIKELIHOOD RATIO FUNCTION
C
40       WRITE(4,710)
         SUMP=0.D0
         DO 9 I=1,KG
         READ(5,506)PRIOR(I)
9        SUMP=SUMP+PRIOR(I)
         IF(SUMP.EQ.1.D0.OR.SUMP.EQ.2.D0)GOTO12
         WRITE(4,712)
         GOTO40
C
C          ITYP=0, MIXTURE SAMPLING SCHEME. COMPUTE PRIORS.
C
10       DO 11 I=1,KG
11       PRIOR(I)=DFLOAT(N(I))/NOBS
12       CONTINUE
C
13       CONTINUE
C
C          LOOP ON THE VARIABLES USED IN THE LOGISTIC DISCRIMINANT
C          ANALYSIS. CHOOSE AMONG THE NV VARIABLES. GIVE NUMBER OF
C          VARIABLES (NVAR) AND THEIR CODES (LIST).
C
C          TO STOP PROGRAM, SET NVAR=0.
C
         WRITE(4,711)
         READ(5,508)NVAR,(LIST(I),I=1,NVAR)
         IF(NVAR.EQ.0)GOTO100
         WRITE(4,709)
         READ(5,505)ISDX
C
C          COMPUTE GROUP AND OVERALL MEANS AND STANDARD DEVIATIONS FOR ALL
C          NVAR VARIABLES SELECTED. LOOK FOR DATA NEEDED IN VECTOR Y AND
C          STORE IN A NEW VECTOR X TO BE USED IN THE SUBROUTINE.
C
         NTOT=0
         K=0
         L=2
         MTOT=N(1)
         JG=1
         JGT=1
         NT(JG)=0
         DO 15 I=1,NOBS
         KK=(I-1)*NV1+1
         K=K+1
         X(K)=Y(KK)
         DO 14 J=1,NVAR
         K=K+1
14       X(K)=Y(KK+LIST(J))
C
C          OVERALL MEANS AND SDS
C
```

```
      CALL LOGIO8(X(L),NVAR,LISTX,1.DO,NTOT,TW,XBAR,SD)
C
C       GROUP MEANS AND SDS
C
      CALL LOGIO8(X(L),NVAR,LISTX,1.DO,NT(JG),TWT(JG),
     *            XB(JGT),STD(JGT))
      IF(I.LT.MTOT)GOTO42
      JG=JG+1
      NT(JG)=0
      JGT=JGT+NVAR
      MTOT=MTOT+N(JG)
42    CONTINUE
      L=L+NVAR+1
15    CONTINUE
      DF=NTOT-1
      LISTC(1)=0
      DO 16 J=1,NVAR
      JJ=J+1
      LISTC(JJ)=J
16    SD(J)=DSQRT(SD(J)/DF)
      DO 43 J=1,KG
      JM=(J-1)*NVAR
      DF=N(J)-1
      DO 43 JJ=1,NVAR
      JL=JM+JJ
43    STD(JL)=DSQRT(STD(JL)/DF)
      NVAR1=NVAR+1
      NB=KG1*NVAR1
      DO 17 J=1,NB
17    B(J)=0.DO
      IF(ISDX.EQ.0)GOTO20
C
C       ISDX=1, STANDARDIZE DATA MATRIX.
C
      L=1
      DO 19 I=1,NOBS
      DO 18 J=1,NVAR
      L=L+1
18    X(L)=(X(L)-XBAR(J))/SD(J)
19    L=L+1
20    CONTINUE
C
C       PRINT RESULTS.
C
      WRITE(6,600)DAY,HOUR
      DO 21 I=1,KG
21    WRITE(6,601)I,N(I),PRIOR(I),(GNAME(J,I),J=1,20)
      WRITE(6,602)NOBS
      WRITE(6,603)
      WRITE(6,604)
      DO 22 J=1,NVAR
22    WRITE(6,605)LIST(J),XBAR(J),SD(J),(XNAME(JJ,LIST(J)),JJ=1,20)
```

```
C
      WRITE(6,620)
      CALL LOGIO6(XB,NVAR,KG,6,LISTG,LIST)
      WRITE(6,621)
      CALL LOGIO6(STD,NVAR,KG,6,LISTG,LIST)
C
      WRITE(6,606)FILE,FMT
C
C       PERFORM LOGISTIC DISCRIMINANT ANALYSIS: ML ESTIMATION
C
      CALL LOGMLE(X,NVAR,N,KG,ISDX,ITYP,PRIOR,CYCLE,B)
      WRITE(6,622)DAY,HOUR
C
C       IF ISDX=1, TRANSFORM MATRIX OF COEFFICIENTS TO ORIGINAL DATA.
C
      IF(ISDX.EQ.0)GOTO25
      L=0
      DO 24 I=1,KG1
      L=L+1
      SUM=0.DO
      DO 23 J=1,NVAR
      L=L+1
      BC(L)=B(L)/SD(J)
23    SUM=SUM+BC(L)*XBAR(J)
      LL=NVAR1*(I-1)+1
24    BC(LL)=B(LL)-SUM
      WRITE(6,613)
      CALL LOGIO6(BC,NVAR1,KG1,6,LISTG,LISTC)
25    CONTINUE
C
C       IF IDATA=0, PRINT ALL RESULTS
C       IF IDATA=1, SKIP TO NEXT PROBLEM
C
      IF(IDATA.EQ.1)GOTO13
C
C       PRINT GROUP PROBABILITIES FOR EACH PATIENT.
C
      WRITE(6,607)
      WRITE(6,608)(LISTG(J),J=1,KG)
      JG=1
      ISUM=N(1)
      K=1
      WRITE(6,609)
      DO 30 I=1,NOBS
      IF(I.LE.ISUM)GOTO26
      JG=JG+1
      ISUM=ISUM+N(JG)
      WRITE(6,609)
26    CONTINUE
      KK=1
      DO 27 IS=1,KG1
      CALL LOGIO1(B(KK),1,NVAR1,X(K),1,KSI(IS))
```

```
27      KK=KK+NVAR1
        CALL LOGPRO(KSI,PSI,KG)
        PSIMAX=0.D0
        DO 29 IS=1,KG
        IF(PSI(IS).LE.PSIMAX)GOTO29
        MAX=IS
        PSIMAX=PSI(IS)
29      CONTINUE
        WRITE(6,610)I,NPAT(I),JG,MAX,(PSI(J),J=1,KG)
        K=K+NVAR1
30      CONTINUE
C
C         PRINT MATRIX OF OBSERVATIONS.
C
        WRITE(6,611)(LIST(J),J=1,NVAR)
        WRITE(6,609)
        JG=1
        ISUM=N(1)
        J1=2
        J2=NVAR1
        DO 32 I=1,NOBS
        IF(I.LE.ISUM)GOTO31
        JG=JG+1
        ISUM=ISUM+N(JG)
        WRITE(6,609)
31      CONTINUE
        WRITE(6,612)I,NPAT(I),JG,(X(J),J=J1,J2)
        J1=J1+NVAR1
        J2=J1+NVAR-1
32      CONTINUE
33      CONTINUE
C
C         PRINT MATRIX OF SCORES. REMEMBER THAT, IF KG IS THE NUMBER
C         OF GROUPS, THERE ARE KG1=KG-1 SCORES FOR EACH SUBJECT!!
C         THESE SCORES ENABLE TO ALLOCATE THE SUBJECT AND TO COMPUTE
C         THE PROBABILITY OF BELONGING TO EACH GROUP.
C
        WRITE(6,614)(LISTG(J),J=1,KG1)
        JG=1
        ISUM=N(1)
        K=1
        WRITE(6,609)
        DO 36 I=1,NOBS
        IF(I.LE.ISUM)GOTO34
        JG=JG+1
        ISUM=ISUM+N(JG)
        WRITE(6,609)
34      CONTINUE
        KK=1
        DO 35 IS=1,KG1
        KSI(IS)=0.D0
        CALL LOGI01(B(KK),1,NVAR1,X(K),1,KSI(IS))
```

```
 35     KK=KK+NVAR1
        WRITE(6,612)I,NPAT(I),JG,(KSI(J),J=1,KG1)
        K=K+NVAR1
 36     CONTINUE
C
C         IF NEW PROBLEM, READ NVAR AND LIST. OTHERWISE, EXIT.
C
        GOTO13
100     STOP
C
500     FORMAT(20A1)
501     FORMAT(I2)
502     FORMAT(20A4)
503     FORMAT(10A8)
504     FORMAT(6I3)
505     FORMAT(I1)
506     FORMAT(F10.0)
508     FORMAT(40I2)
C
600     FORMAT(//1H1,'MULTIPLE GROUP LOGISTIC DISCRIMINANT',
     *         ' ANALYSIS'/1X,45(1H*)//1X,'DATE ... ',9A1/
     *         1X,'TIME ... ',8A1//1X,'OUTPUT FROM MAIN',
     *         ' PROGRAM - L O G D I S '////
     *         3X,'DISCRIMINATION BETWEEN:'/3X,23(1H*)/)
601     FORMAT(8X,'GROUP:',I2,3X,'N=',I3,5X,'PRIOR=',F5.2,5X,20A4)
602     FORMAT(/8X,'TOTAL NO. OF OBSERVATIONS =',I4)
603     FORMAT(//3X,'VARIABLES STUDIED'/3X,17(1H*)/)
604     FORMAT(8X,'NUMBER',3X,'OVERALL MEAN',4X,'OVERALL S.D.',5X,
     *         'NAME'/)
605     FORMAT(10X,I2,7X,F10.2,6X,F10.3,5X,20A4)
606     FORMAT(////1X,'DATABASE INFORMATION'/1X,20(1H*)//
     *         1X,'FILE NAME = ',20A1/1X,'FORMAT USED = ',10A8)
607     FORMAT(1H1//3X,'MATRIX OF ALLOCATION AND PROBABILITIES'
     *         /3X,38(1H*))
608     FORMAT(/3X,'I',2X,'NPAT',6X,'GROUP',8X,'GROUP PROB'/13X,'TRUE',
     *         3X,'ALLOC',5X,I1,9I10/)
609     FORMAT(/)
610     FORMAT(1X,I3,2X,A4,5X,I1,6X,I1,10F10.2)
611     FORMAT(1H1//3X,'MATRIX OF OBSERVATIONS'/3X,22(1H*)//3X,'I',2X,
     *  'NPAT',6X,'GROUP',5X,'VAR',2X,I3,9I10,2(/17X,10I10))
612     FORMAT(1X,I3,2X,A4,8X,I1,5X,10F10.2,2(/17X,10F10.2))
613     FORMAT(//5X,'ISDX=1: ORIGINAL MATRIX OF COEFFICIENTS'/5X,
     *         39(1H*)/)
614     FORMAT(1H1//3X,'MATRIX OF SCORES'/3X,16(1H*)//3X,'I',2X,
     *         'NPAT',6X,'GROUP',4X,'SCORES',I3,9I10)
620     FORMAT(///3X,'MATRIX OF MEAN VALUES'/3X,21(1H*)/6X,
     *         'COLUMNS=GROUPS'/6X,'ROWS=VARIABLES')
621     FORMAT(//3X,'MATRIX OF STANDARD DEVIATIONS'/3X,29(1H*)/10X,
     *         'COLUMNS=GROUPS'/10X,'ROWS=VARIABLES')
622     FORMAT(///3X,'DATE ... ',9A1/3X,'TIME ... ',8A1)
C
700     FORMAT(//5X,'READ FILENAME................20A1'/)
```

```
701     FORMAT(/5X,'READ TOTAL NO. OF GROUPS (KG)...I2')
702     FORMAT(/5X,'READ NAME OF EACH GROUP..ONE/LINE...80 CHAR MAX')
703     FORMAT(/5X,'READ TOTAL NO. OF VARIABLES (NV)....I2')
704     FORMAT(/5X,'READ NAME OF THE NV VARIABLES...ONE/LINE..80CH MAX')
705     FORMAT(//5X,'READ DATA FORMAT...NPAT(A),NGROUP(I),DATA(F)'/)
706     FORMAT(/5X,'READ NO. AND ACCEPTED CODES FOR GROUP:',I1,'..5I3')
707     FORMAT(/5X,'DO YOU WANT DATA MATRIX+SCORES?..YES=0,NO=1..I1'/)
708     FORMAT(/5X,'IF MIXTURE SAMPLING, TYPE 0'/5X,
     *          'IF SEPARATE SAMPLING, TYPE 1')
709     FORMAT(/5X,'DO YOU WANT TO WORK WITH THE STANDARDIZED DATA'
     *    ,' MATRIX?'/5X,'NO=0, YES=1.....I1'/)
710     FORMAT(/5X,'SEPARATE SAMPLING SCHEME SELECTED'/
     *       5X,'ENTER PRIOR PROB FOR EACH GROUP....ONE/LINE..F10.0')
711     FORMAT(/5X,'ENTER NO. OF VARIABLES AND THEIR CODES...40I2'/)
712     FORMAT(/5X,'PRIORS DO NOT SUM UP TO 1!!...REENTER')
713     FORMAT(//3X,'WARNING MESSAGE: ',I5,' VALUES HAVE BEEN STORED',
     *          ' IN VECTOR Y.'/3X,'HAS THIS VECTOR BE PROPERLY',
     *          ' DIMENSIONED ?  IF NOT, PROBLEMS !')
C
        END


        SUBROUTINE LOGMLE(X,NVAR,N,KG,ISDX,ITYP,PRIOR,CYCLE,B)
C       *****************************************************
C
C         SUBROUTINE COMPUTING THE MAXIMUM LIKELIHOOD ESTIMATES (MLE)
C         OF THE COEFFICIENTS OF THE LOGISTIC DISCRIMINANT FUNCTIONS
C         BETWEEN KG GROUPS.
C
C         MLE ARE OBTAINED USING THE NEWTON-RAPHSON ITERATIVE PROCEDURE
C
C         VERSION: January 1986
C
C         X:      MATRIX OF OBSERVATIONS STORED IN ONE-DIMENSIONAL VECTOR
C                 MULTIVARIATE OBSERVATIONS ARE ORDERED BY GROUP.
C                 DIMENSION OF X IS NVAR*(N(1)+...+N(KG)).
C         NVAR:   NUMBER OF VARIABLES
C         N:      VECTOR OF LENGTH KG CONTAINING THE NUMBER OF OBSERVATIONS
C                 OF EACH GROUP.
C         KG:     NUMBER OF GROUPS
C         ISDX:   INDICATES WHETHER THE DATA MATRIX HAS BEEN STANDARDIZED
C                 (ISDX=1) OR NOT (ISDX=0).
C         ITYP:   INDICATES TYPE OF SAMPLING. MIXTURE SAMPLING (ITYP=0),
C                 SEPARATE SAMPLING (ITYP=1).
C         PRIOR:  VECTOR OF LENGTH KG CONTAINING THE PRIOR PROBABILITIES
C                 OF THE KG GROUPS. IF ITYP=0, PRIOR(I)=N(I)/NOBS,
C                 WHERE NOBS=N(1)+...+N(KG). IF ITYP=1, THE PRIORS ARE
C                 SUPPLIED BY THE USER.
C         CYCLE:  INTEGER GIVING THE FREQUENCY WITH WHICH THE HESSIAN
C                 MATRIX SHOULD BE UPDATED. HAS BEEN SET EQUAL TO 1.
C         B:      ON INPUT, CONTAINS THE INITIAL VALUES OF THE COEFFICIENTS
C                 OF THE DISCRIMINANT FUNCTIONS (USUALLY ZEROS)
```

```
C                 ON OUTPUT, CONTAINS THE MLE OF THE COEFFICIENTS.
C                 THE LENGTH OF VECTOR B IS (NVAR+1)*(KG-1).
C
C          ROUTINES CALLED: LOGIO1, LOGIO2, LOGIO3, LOGIO4,
C                           LOGIO5, LOGIO6, INDICE, LOGPRO
C
C          THE SUBROUTINE IS ABLE TO DETECT COMPLETE AND QUASI-COMPLETE
C          SEPARATION IN THE DATA SET, CONDITIONS FOR WHICH THE MLE
C          ARE INFINITE AND THEREFORE DO NOT EXIST.
C
C          IF NV1=NVAR+1, KG1=KG-1, NK=NV1*KG1, NNK=NK*(NK+1)/2, THEN
C          WE HAVE THE FOLLOWING DIMENSIONS: (HERE NVAR=10,KG=5)
C
C          C(NK),WORK(NK),BB(NK),DB(NK),SEB(NK),ZB(NK),LISTH(NK),H(NNK),
C          PSI(KG),KSI(KG),ERR(KG,KG),LISTR(NV1),LISTC(KG).
C
C***********************************************************************
C
      IMPLICIT REAL*8(A-H,O-Z)
      REAL*8 KSI(5)
      DIMENSION X(1),B(1),C(44),H(990),WORK(44),BB(44),DB(44),PSI(5)
      DIMENSION SEB(44),ZB(44),PRIOR(1)
      INTEGER CYCLE,ERR(5,5),CIT,CITIT,LISTH(44),N(1),T,TJ,T1
      INTEGER LISTR(11),LISTC(5)
      LOGICAL SEPLDF,MAXLDF,FINLDF,INVLDF,QCSLDF
      COMMON/RESULT/ERR,ISEP,IQSEP,IWARN,IERROR,CITIT,RLL1
C
C          INITIALIZATIONS.
C
      EPSI=1.D-6
      IWARN=0
      HMAX=1000.D0
      ISEP=0
      IQSEP=0
      IERROR=0
      INV=0
      CIT=0
      IT=0
      KG1=KG-1
      NOBS=0
      RLLO=0.D0
      DO 1 I=1,KG
      LISTC(I)=I
      RLLO=RLLO+N(I)*DLOG(DFLOAT(N(I)))
1     NOBS=NOBS+N(I)
      RLLO=RLLO-NOBS*DLOG(DFLOAT(NOBS))
      NVAR1=NVAR+1
      NC=KG1*NVAR1
      MM=NC*(NC+1)/2
      L=0
      DO 2 I=1,KG1
      DO 2 J=1,NVAR1
```

```
      L=L+1
2     LISTH(L)=10*I+J-1
      DO 3 J=1,NVAR1
3     LISTR(J)=J-1
      RLL=-1.D10
      RLMAX=-1.D10
      SEPLDF=.FALSE.
      QCSLDF=.FALSE.
      MAXLDF=.FALSE.
      FINLDF=.FALSE.
      EPS=1.D-6
C
C       PRINT PARAMETERS OF THE PROBLEM.
C
      WRITE(6,600)KG,NVAR,NOBS,CYCLE
      DO 4 I=1,KG
4     WRITE(6,601)I,N(I),PRIOR(I)
      IF(ITYP.EQ.0)GOTO5
      WRITE(6,602)ITYP
C
C       CHECK WHETHER USER RUNS THE PROGRAM LOGISD
C       FOR CALCULATING A LIKELIHOOD RATIO FUNCTION.
C
      XLR=PRIOR(1)+PRIOR(2)
      IF(XLR.NE.2)GOTO6
      WRITE(6,627)
      GOTO6
5     WRITE(6,603)ITYP
6     CONTINUE
C
      IF(ISDX.EQ.0)GOTO7
      WRITE(6,604)ISDX
      GOTO8
7     WRITE(6,605)ISDX
8     CONTINUE
C
C       START THE NEWTON-RAPHSON ITERATIVE PROCEDURE.
C
9     CONTINUE
      IF(FINLDF.OR.CIT.EQ.0)GOTO10
      GOTO22
10    CITIT=IT+CIT
      WRITE(6,606)CITIT,INV
      IF(FINLDF)GOTO11
      WRITE(6,607)
      CALL LOGI06(B,NVAR1,KG1,6,LISTC,LISTR)
      WRITE(6,608)
      GOTO21
C
C       PROCESS HAS REACHED MAXIMUM OF LIKELIHOOD FUNCTION.
C
11    CONTINUE
```

```
      IF(ITYP.EQ.0.OR.SEPLDF.OR.QCSLDF)GOTO20
C
C       SEPARATE SAMPLING SCHEME. ADJUST FOR CHANGES IN PRIORS.
C
      DO 12 T=1,KG
      DO 12 T1=1,KG
12    ERR(T,T1)=0
      KK=1
      DO 13 I=1,KG1
      B(KK)=B(KK)+DLOG(N(KG)*PRIOR(I))-DLOG(N(I)*PRIOR(KG))
13    KK=KK+NVAR1
      DO 14 T=1,KG1
      K=(T-1)*NVAR1
      K=K*(K+1)/2
      FACT=1.D0
      DO 14 T1=1,T
      IF(T.EQ.T1)FACT=1.D0+DFLOAT(N(KG))/N(T)
      KK=K+(T1-1)*NVAR1+1
14    H(KK)=H(KK)-FACT/N(KG)
C
C       COMPUTE FINAL ALLOCATION MATRIX.
C
      K=1
      JG=1
      ISUM=N(1)
      DO 19 I=1,NOBS
      IF(I.LE.ISUM)GOTO15
      JG=JG+1
      ISUM=ISUM+N(JG)
15    CONTINUE
      KK=1
      DO 16 IS=1,KG1
      CALL LOGI01(B(KK),1,NVAR1,X(K),1,KSI(IS))
16    KK=KK+NVAR1
      CALL LOGPRO(KSI,PSI,KG)
      PSIMAX=0.D0
      DO 18 IS=1,KG
      IF(PSI(IS).LE.PSIMAX)GOTO18
      MAX=IS
      PSIMAX=PSI(IS)
18    CONTINUE
      ERR(JG,MAX)=ERR(JG,MAX)+1
19    K=K+NVAR1
20    CONTINUE
      WRITE(6,609)
      CALL LOGI06(B,NVAR1,KG1,6,LISTC,LISTR)
21    WRITE(6,610)
22    IF(FINLDF)GOTO23
      GOTO26
C
C       AT LAST ITERATION, PRINT MATRICES OF ESTIMATED COEFFICIENTS,
C       STANDARD-ERRORS OF COEFFICIENTS, Z-SCORES AND ASYMPTOTIC
```

```
C          DISPERSION MATRIX OF COEFFICIENTS. ALSO PRINT THE FINAL
C          ALLOCATION MATRIX.
C
23       CONTINUE
         DO 24 I=1,NC
         II=I
         J=INDICE(II,II)
         SEB(I)=DSQRT(H(J))
24       ZB(I)=B(I)/SEB(I)
         WRITE(6,611)
         CALL LOGIO6(SEB,NVAR1,KG1,6,LISTC,LISTR)
         WRITE(6,612)
         CALL LOGIO6(ZB,NVAR1,KG1,6,LISTC,LISTR)
         WRITE(6,613)
         CALL LOGIO5(H,NC,LISTH,6)
         WRITE(6,614)(LISTC(I),I=1,KG)
         WRITE(6,610)
         DO 25 I=1,KG
25       WRITE(6,615)I,(ERR(J,I),J=1,KG)
         WRITE(6,616)(N(I),I=1,KG)
C
C          COMPUTE DISCRIMINANT EFFECTIVENESS OF THE VECTOR
C          USING AN ASYMPTOTIC CHI-SQUARE CRITERION (NVAR DF).
C
         CHI2=2*(RLL1-RLLO)
         IDFCHI=KG1*NVAR
         PROCHI=PRCHI2(CHI2,IDFCHI,IFAULT)
         WRITE(6,626)CHI2,IDFCHI,PROCHI
         GOTO100
26       CONTINUE
         IF(CIT.GT.25)GOTO27
         GOTO28
C
C          NO CONVERGENCE AFTER 25 ITERATIONS. STOP PROCESS.
C
27       WRITE(6,617)
         CALL LOGIO6(BB,NVAR1,KG1,6,LISTC,LISTR)
         IERROR=3
         GOTO100
C
C          NEW ITERATION OF THE PROCESS. REINITIALIZE SOME ELEMENTS.
C
28       RLL1=RLL
         DO 29 I=1,KG
         DO 29 J=1,KG
29       ERR(I,J)=0
         PRBMAX=0.DO
         ISEPA=1
         RLL=0.DO
         CIT=CIT+1
         INVLDF=.FALSE.
         DO 30 I=1,NC
```

```
 30     C(I)=0.D0
        IF(CIT-(CIT/CYCLE)*CYCLE.EQ.1.OR.CYCLE.EQ.1)GOTO31
        GOTO33
 31     INVLDF=.TRUE.
        DO 32 I=1,MM
 32     H(I)=0.D0
 33     CONTINUE
C
C         COMPUTE LOG-LIKELIHOOD, GRADIENT VECTOR, HESSIAN MATRIX,
C         AND CLASSIFICATION MATRIX.
C
        K=1
        JG=1
        ISUM=N(1)
        DO 45 I=1,NOBS
        IF(I.LE.ISUM)GOTO34
        JG=JG+1
        ISUM=ISUM+N(JG)
 34     CONTINUE
        KK=1
C
C         COMPUTE THE PROBABILITY FOR THE I-TH SUBJECT IN ALL GROUPS.
C
        DO 35 IS=1,KG1
        CALL LOGI01(B(KK),1,NVAR1,X(K),1,KSI(IS))
 35     KK=KK+NVAR1
        CALL LOGPRO(KSI,PSI,KG)
C
C         COMPUTE CONTRIBUTION TO LOG-LIKELIHOOD (RLL).
C
        RLL=RLL+DLOG(PSI(JG))
C
C         COMPUTE CONTRIBUTION TO GRADIENT VECTOR (C).
C
        DO 37 T=1,KG1
        DO 37 J=1,NVAR1
        KJ=K+J-1
        JT=(T-1)*NVAR1+J
        C(JT)=C(JT)-PSI(T)*X(KJ)
        IF(T.EQ.JG)C(JT)=C(JT)+X(KJ)
 37     CONTINUE
        IF(INVLDF)GOTO38
        GOTO41
C
C         COMPUTE CONTRIBUTION TO HESSIAN MATRIX (H).
C
 38     DO 40 T=1,KG1
        DO 40 T1=1,T
        DO 40 J=1,NVAR1
        KJ=K+J-1
        IR=(T-1)*NVAR1+J
        JJ1=NVAR1
```

```
      FACT=PSI(T)*PSI(T1)*X(KJ)
      IF(T.NE.T1)GOTO39
      JJ1=J
      FACT=-PSI(T)*(1.D0-PSI(T))*X(KJ)
39    CONTINUE
      DO 40 J1=1,JJ1
      KJ1=K+J1-1
      IR1=(T1-1)*NVAR1+J1
      IRR1=INDICE(IR,IR1)
      H(IRR1)=H(IRR1)-FACT*X(KJ1)
40    CONTINUE
C
C       CLASSIFICATION MATRIX UPDATE (ERR).
C
41    PSIMAX=0.D0
      DO 42 IS=1,KG
      IF(PSI(IS).LE.PSIMAX)GOTO42
      MAX=IS
      PSIMAX=PSI(IS)
42    CONTINUE
      ERR(JG,MAX)=ERR(JG,MAX)+1
C
C       IS THE CURRENT OBSERVATION CORRECTLY ALLOCATED?
C
43    IF(MAX.NE.JG)ISEPA=0
C
C       FIND LARGEST CORRECT PROBABILITY ACROSS SAMPLE.
C
44    IF(CIT.GT.1.AND.PSI(JG).GT.PRBMAX)PRBMAX=PSI(JG)
C
45    K=K+NVAR1
C
      WRITE(6,618)CIT,RLL
      IF(.NOT.MAXLDF.AND.RLL.LT.RLL1)GOTO46
      GOTO47
46    MAXLDF=.TRUE.
      RLMAX=RLL1
47    IF(MAXLDF.AND.RLL.GT.RLMAX)MAXLDF=.FALSE.
      IF(CIT.EQ.1)GOTO54
C
C       IS THERE COMPLETE SEPARATION IN THE DATA SET?
C       IF SO, MLE ARE KNOWN NOT TO EXIST. STOP PROCESS.
C
      IF(ISEPA.EQ.1)GOTO51
C
C       IS THERE QUASI-COMPLETE SEPARATION?
C       IF SO, MLE ARE KNOWN NOT TO EXIST. PRINT WARNING MESSAGE.
C       THIS TEST APPLIES IF ISDX=0 AND AFTER AT LEAST 7 ITERATIONS.
C
      IF(ISDX.EQ.1.OR.IWARN.EQ.1)GOTO54
      IF(CIT.LT.8)GOTO48
      IF(PRBMAX.GT.PRBQCS)GOTO66
```

```
48      EPS1=1.DO-PRBMAX
        IF(EPSI.GT.EPS1)EPSI=EPS1
        PRBQCS=1.DO-EPSI
        GOTO54
50      CONTINUE
        QCSLDF=.TRUE.
        IQSEP=1
        GOTO52
51      WRITE(6,620)
        SEPLDF=.TRUE.
        ISEP=1
52      IF(.NOT.INVLDF)GOTO53
        INV=INV+1
        CALL LOGIO3(H,NC,H,WORK,NULL,IFAULT)
53      FINLDF=.TRUE.
        WRITE(6,621)
        GOTO9
54      IF(INVLDF)GOTO55
        GOTO58
55      CONTINUE
        CALL LOGIO3(H,NC,H,WORK,NULL,IFAULT)
        IF(IFAULT.GT.O)GOTO65
C
C         SECOND CHECK FOR QUASI-COMPLETE SEPARATION BASED ON THE
C         DIAGONAL ELEMENTS OF THE ASYMPTOTIC DISPERSION MATRIX.
C         THIS TEST APPLIES ONLY IF ISDX=1!
C
        IF(ISDX.EQ.0)GOTO57
        DO 56 J=1,NC
        JJ=J
        L=INDICE(JJ,JJ)
        IF(H(L).LT.HMAX)GOTO56
        WRITE(6,622)J,H(L)
        IQSEP=1
        QCSLDF=.TRUE.
        GOTO53
56      CONTINUE
57      CONTINUE
        INV=INV+1
C
C         HAS THE MAXIMUM OF THE LIKELIHOOD FUNCTION BEEN ATTAINED?
C
58      IF(DABS((RLL-RLL1)/RLL1).LT.EPS)GOTO59
        GOTO60
C
C         YES, MAXIMUM ATTAINED!
C
59      WRITE(6,623)CIT,RLL1
        IT=IT+CIT
        CIT=0
        IF(INVLDF)FINLDF=.TRUE.
        GOTO9
```

```
 60      IF(.NOT.MAXLDF)GOTO61
         GOTO63
C
C          NO, NOT MAXIMUM YET!
C
 61      DO 62 I=1,NC
 62      BB(I)=B(I)
 63      CALL LOGI04(H,NC,C,DB)
         DO 64 I=1,NC
 64      B(I)=B(I)+DB(I)
         GOTO9
C
C          THE HESSIAN MATRIX IS SINGULAR, STOP PROCESS.
C
 65      WRITE(6,624)
         IERROR=1
         GOTO100
 66      IWARN=1
         WRITE(6,625)
         GOTO54
100      RETURN
C
C
600      FORMAT(1H1//3X,'LOGISTIC DISCRIMINANT ANALYSIS'/3X,'MAXIMUM',
     *   ' LIKELIHOOD ESTIMATION'/3X,29(1H*)//3X,'PARAMETERS',
     *   ' OF THE PROBLEM'//3X,'NO. OF GROUPS =',I2,5X,'NO. OF VARIABLES'
     *   ,' =',I3,5X,'TOTAL NO. OF OBS =',I3/3X,'H-INV CYCLE =',I2//)
601      FORMAT(3X,'GROUP ',I1,5X,'N = ',I3,5X,'PRIOR = ',F4.2)
602      FORMAT(//3X,'ITYP = ',I1,': SEPARATE SAMPLING SCHEME'/
     *   13X,'PRIORS ARE GIVEN BY USER'/13X,'ADJUSTMENT OF MLE REQUIRED',
     *      ' FOR INDEPENDENT TERMS'/)
603      FORMAT(//3X,'ITYP = ',I1,': MIXTURE SAMPLING SCHEME'/
     *     13X,'PRIORS ARE COMPUTED FROM THE SAMPLE'/)
604      FORMAT(//3X,'ISDX = ',I1,': STANDARDIZED MATRIX OF DATA'//)
605      FORMAT(//3X,'ISDX = ',I1,': ORIGINAL MATRIX OF DATA'//)
606      FORMAT(//3X,'ITERATION',I3,3X,'INVERSION',I3)
607      FORMAT(/3X,'INITIAL MATRIX OF COEFFICIENTS B')
608      FORMAT(//3X,'NEWTON-RAPHSON ITERATIVE PROCEDURE')
609      FORMAT(/3X,'FINAL MATRIX OF COEFFICIENTS B')
610      FORMAT(/)
611      FORMAT(/3X,'MATRIX OF STD-ERRORS OF COEFFICIENTS SEB')
612      FORMAT(//3X,'MATRIX OF Z-SCORES: ZB=B/SEB')
613      FORMAT(//3X,'ASYMPTOTIC DISPERSION MATRIX OF COEFFICIENTS')
614      FORMAT(///3X,'FINAL CLASSIFICATION MATRIX OF OBSERVATIONS'/15X,
     *       'COLUMNS=TRUE GROUPS'/15X,'ROWS=ALLOCATED GROUPS'//8X,10I8)
615      FORMAT(6X,I2,10I8)
616      FORMAT(/5X,'TOTAL',I6,9I8)
617      FORMAT(3X,'PROCESS STOPPED AFTER 25 ITERATIONS...RERUN'//
     *    3X,'CURRENT MATRIX OF COEFFICIENTS'//)
618      FORMAT(3X,'IT =',I3,3X,'LOG-LIK =',F12.6)
620      FORMAT(//3X,'COMPLETE SEPARATION IN THE DATA SET')
621      FORMAT(/3X,'IT IS KNOWN THAT THE ML ESTIMATORS DO NOT EXIST'/
```

```
     *    3X,'THE COEFFICIENTS ARE QUITE ARBITRARY'/3X,'THE ASYMPTOTIC',
     *      ' DISPERSION MATRIX BLOWS UP!'/3X,'THE CLASSIFICATION',
     *      ' MATRIX IS CORRECT'//)
622   FORMAT(//3X,'QUASI-COMPLETE SEPARATION HIGHLY SUSPECTED'/3X,
     *    'ONE DIAGONAL ELEMENT OF THE DISPERSION MATRIX IS TOO LARGE:'
     *    ,' H(',I2,') = ',F7.1/)
623   FORMAT(/3X,'MAXIMUM ATTAINED AFTER',I3,' ITERATIONS:  MAX LOG-'
     *           ,'LIK =', F12.6/)
624   FORMAT(//3X,'HESSIAN MATRIX IS SINGULAR - PROCESS STOPPED')
625   FORMAT(/5X,'WARNING MESSAGE:QUASI-COMPLETE SEPARATION SUSPECTED'
     *   ,' IN THE DATASET'/5X,'TO HAVE A CONFIRMATION, RUN THE PROGRAM'
     *   ,' ON THE STANDARDIZED DATA (ISDX=1).'/5X,'CHECK WHETHER SOME'
     *   ,' DIAGONAL ELEMENTS OF THE HESSIAN MATRIX BLOW UP.'/5X,
     *   'IF SO, THERE IS QUASI-COMPLETE SEPARATION IN THE DATASET.',
     *   ' IF NOT, THERE IS'/5X,'OVERLAP, MLE EXIST AND ARE UNIQUE:',
     *   ' THE WARNING INDICATES THAT THERE'/5X,'IS AT LEAST OBSERV'
     *   ,'ATION CORRECTLY ALLOCATED WITH A PROBABILITY EXTREMELY'
     *   /5X,'CLOSE TO 1 (ATYPICAL OBSERVATION).'//)
626   FORMAT(///3X,'EFFECTIVENESS - CHI-SQUARE:',F8.2,3X,'DF:',I3,
     *         3X,'PROB:',D12.4)
627   FORMAT(//3X,'ATTENTION: BOTH PRIORS ARE EQUAL TO ONE'/
     *    3X,9(1H*)//7X,'- PROGRAM "LOGISD" IS USED FOR COMPUTING'/
     *    9X,'THE LIKELIHOOD RATIO FUNCTION BETWEEN'/
     *    9X,'GROUP1 (D) AND GROUP2 (DBAR):'//
     *    17X,'L(X) = EXP(BO + B.X)'//9X,'WHERE BO AND B ARE GIVEN IN',
     *    ' FINAL MATRIX'/9X,'OF COEFFICIENTS B BELOW'//7X,'- IN',
     *    ' THE CLASSIFICATION MATRIX BELOW,'/9X,'COLUMNS ARE GROUPS ',
     *    'D AND DBAR, WHILE'/9X,'ROWS ARE L>1 AND L<1, RESPECTIVELY'/)
C
      END




      SUBROUTINE LOGPRO(KSI,PSI,KG)
C     *****************************
C
C       CALCULATES POSTERIOR PROBABILITIES (PSI) FROM SCORE VECTOR (KSI)
C       UNDER THE KG-GROUP LOGISTIC DISCRIMINATION MODEL. WORK IS A
C       WORKING ARRAY OF LENGTH KG AT LEAST.
C
C       THIS ROUTINE IS SPECIALLY DESIGNED TO AVOID UNDERFLOWS OR
C       OVERFLOWS WHEN COMPUTING THE PROBABILITIES WITH THE USE OF
C       THE EXPONENTIAL FUNCTION. "CONST" IS A CONSTANT, WHICH IS
C       MACHINE DEPENDENT AND SHOULD BE CHANGED APPROPRIATELY BY USER.
C
      IMPLICIT REAL*8(A-H,O-Z)
      REAL*8 KSI(1),PSI(1),WORK(10)
C
      CONST=50.0D0
```

```
      KSI(KG)=0.DO
      DO 3 IS=1,KG
      PSI(IS)=0.DO
      DO 1 IT=1,KG
      WORK(IT)=KSI(IT)-KSI(IS)
C
C       ACTION AGAINST UNDER- OR OVER-FLOW
C
      ADIF=DABS(WORK(IT))
      IF(ADIF.LT.CONST)GOTO1
      SIGN=WORK(IT)/ADIF
      WORK(IT)=SIGN*(CONST-1.DO)
1     CONTINUE
      DO 2 IT=1,KG
2     PSI(IS)=PSI(IS)+DEXP(WORK(IT))
      PSI(IS)=1.DO/PSI(IS)
3     CONTINUE
      RETURN
      END


      SUBROUTINE LOGIO1(A,NR,NC,B,NCC,C)
C     ********************************
C
C       PRODUCT OF TWO MATRICES HELD IN ONE-DIMENSIONAL FORM.
C       A IS NR*NC, B IS NC*NCC. FORMS C=A*B. C IS NR*NCC.
C
      IMPLICIT REAL*8 (A-H,O-Z)
      DIMENSION A(1),B(1),C(1)
      M=1
      L20=1
      DO 10 I=1,NCC
      L10=1
      DO 11 J=1,NR
      SUM=0.0
      L1=L10
      L2=L20
      DO 12 K=1,NC
      SUM=SUM+A(L1)*B(L2)
      L1=L1+NR
12    L2=L2+1
      C(M)=SUM
      L10=L10+1
11    M=M+1
10    L20=L20+NC
      RETURN
      END
```

```
      SUBROUTINE LOGIO2(A,N,U,NULLTY,IFAULT)
C     ************************************
C
C       ALGORITHM AS 6 J.R.STATIST.SOC C, (1968) VOL.17,NO2.
C       GIVEN A SYMMETRIC MATRIX A(N*N) IN ONE DIMENSIONAL FORM,
C       CALCULATES AN UPPER TRIANGLE SUCH THAT U PRIME*U=A.
C       U IS ALSO HELD IN ONE-DIML. FORM AND MAY COINCIDE WITH A.
C       A MUST BE POSITIVE SEMI-DEFINITE.
C       TOL IS SET TO MULTIPLYING FACTOR DETERMINING EFFECTIVE
C       ZERO FOR PIVOT.
C       NULLTY IS RETURNED AS NO. EFFECTIVE ZERO PIVOTS.
C       IFAULT IS RETURNED AS 1 IF N.LE.0,2 IF A( ) IS NOT POSITIVE
C       SEMI-DEFINITE WITHIN THE TOLERANCE DEFINED BY TOL, OTHERWISE
C       ZERO.
C
      IMPLICIT REAL*8 (A-H,O-Z)
      DIMENSION A(1),U(1)
      DATA TOL/1.0D-10/
      IFAULT=1
      IF(N.LE.0)GOTO100
      IFAULT=2
      NULLTY=0
      J=1
      K=0
      DO 10 ICOL=1,N
      L=0
      DO 11 IROW=1,ICOL
      K=K+1
      W=A(K)
      M=J
      DO 12 I=1,IROW
      L=L+1
      IF(I.EQ.IROW)GOTO13
      UU=U(L)*U(M)
      W=W-UU
12    M=M+1
13    IF(IROW.EQ.ICOL)GOTO14
      IF(U(L).EQ.0.0)GOTO21
16    U(K)=W/U(L)
18    GOTO11
21    U(K)=0.0
      IF(DABS(W).GT.DABS(TOL*A(K)))GOTO100
11    CONTINUE
14    IF(DABS(W).LE.DABS(TOL*A(K)))GOTO20
      IF(W.LT.0.0)GOTO100
      U(K)=DSQRT(W)
      GOTO15
20    U(K)=0.0
      NULLTY=NULLTY+1
15    J=J+ICOL
10    CONTINUE
      IFAULT=0
```

```
100     RETURN
        END


        SUBROUTINE LOGIO3(A,N,C,W,NULLTY,IFAULT)
C       ***************************************
C
C         ALGORITHM AS 7 J.R.STATIST.SOC.C,(1968) VOL.17,NO 2.
C         FORMS IN C( ) AS LOWER TRIANGLE, A GENERALISED INVERSE
C         OF THE POSITIVE SEMI-DEFINITE SYMMETRIC MATRIX A( )
C         ORDER N,STORED AS LOWER TRIANGLE.
C         C( ) MAY COINCIDE WITH A( ). NULLTY IS RETURNED AS THE NULLITY
C         OF A( ). IFAULT IS RETURNED AS 1 IF N.LT.1,2 IF A( ) IS NOT
C         POSITIVE SEMI-DEFINITE, OTHERWISE ZERO.
C         W( ) IS A WORK ARRAY OF LENGTH AT LEAST N THAT IS ALLOCATED BY
C         THE CALLING ROUTINE
C
        IMPLICIT REAL*8(A-H,O-Z)
        DIMENSION A(1),C(1),W(1)
        NROW=N
        IFAULT=1
        IF(NROW.LE.0)GOTO100
        IFAULT=0
        CALL LOGIO2(A,NROW,C,NULLTY,IFAULT)
        IF(IFAULT.NE.0)GOTO100
        NN=N*(N+1)/2
        IROW=N
        NDIAG=NN
16      IF(C(NDIAG).EQ.0.0)GOTO11
        L=NDIAG
        DO 10 I=IROW,N
        W(I)=C(L)
10      L=L+I
        ICOL=N
        JCOL=NN
        MDIAG=NN
15      L=JCOL
        X=0.0
        IF(ICOL.EQ.IROW)X=1.0/W(IROW)
        K=N
13      IF(K.EQ.IROW)GOTO12
        X=X-W(K)*C(L)
        K=K-1
        L=L-1
        IF(L.GT.MDIAG)L=L-K+1
        GOTO13
12      C(L)=X/W(IROW)
        IF(ICOL.EQ.IROW)GOTO14
        MDIAG=MDIAG-ICOL
        ICOL=ICOL-1
        JCOL=JCOL-1
```

```
      GOTO15
11    L=NDIAG
      DO 17 J=IROW,N
      C(L)=0.0
17    L=L+J
14    NDIAG=NDIAG-IROW
      IROW=IROW-1
      IF(IROW.NE.0)GOTO16
100   RETURN
      END


      SUBROUTINE LOGIO4(A,M,B,C)
C     *************************
C
C       PRODUCT OF M-DIMENSIONAL SYMMETRIC MATRIX A BY M-VECTOR B.
C       C=A*B.
C
C       NOTE: C MUST BE DIFFERENT FROM B.
C
      IMPLICIT REAL*8 (A-H,O-Z)
      DIMENSION A(1),B(1),C(1)
      DO 50 I=1,M
      II=(I*(I-1))/2
      SUM=0.0
      IK=II
      DO 15 K=1,I
      IK=IK+1
15    SUM=SUM+A(IK)*B(K)
      IF(I.EQ.M)GOTO50
      IK=II+I
      I1=I+1
      DO 20 K=I1,M
      IK=IK+K-1
20    SUM=SUM+A(IK)*B(K)
50    C(I)=SUM
C
      RETURN
      END


      SUBROUTINE LOGIO5(A,N,LIST,NCHAN)
C     *********************************
C
C       THE SYMMETRIC MATRIX A (N*N) IS OUTPUT ON CHANNEL NCHAN, USING
C       FORMAT F14.4 AND 5 COLUMNS. THE ROWS AND COLUMNS ARE LABELLED
C       WITH THE INTEGERS HELD IN LIST.
C
      IMPLICIT REAL*8(A-H,O-Z)
      DIMENSION A(1),LIST(1)
      DO 10 I=1,N,5
      K1=(I*(I+1))/2
```

```
      K2=K1
      K3=MINO(I+4,N)
      L=0
      WRITE(NCHAN,601)(LIST(K),K=I,K3)
      DO 10 J=I,N
      WRITE(NCHAN,600) LIST(J),(A(K),K=K1,K2)
      K1=K1+J
      IF(L.LT.4)L=L+1
10    K2=K1+L
600   FORMAT(I4,5F14.4)
601   FORMAT(/I15,4I14)
      RETURN
      END


      SUBROUTINE LOGIO6(A,N,M,NCHAN,LISTC,LISTR)
C     ****************************************
C
C       THE MATRIX A(N ROWS * M COLUMNS) IS OUTPUT ON CHANNEL NCHAN,
C       USING FORMAT F14.4 AND 8 COLUMNS. THE ROWS ARE LABELLED WITH
C       THE INTEGERS HELD IN LISTR,AND THE COLUMNS WITH THOSE IN LISTC.
C
      REAL*8 A(1)
      DIMENSION LISTC(1),LISTR(1)
      DO 1 I=1,M,8
      K3=MINO(I+7,M)
      WRITE(NCHAN,601) (LISTC(J),J=I,K3)
      DO 1 J=1,N
1     WRITE(NCHAN,600) LISTR(J),(A((K-1)*N+J),K=I,K3)
600   FORMAT(I4,8F14.4)
601   FORMAT(/I15,7I14)
      RETURN
      END


      SUBROUTINE LOGIO7(X,NVAR,ICHECK)
C     ********************************
C
C       CHECK WHETHER VECTOR X OF LENGTH NVAR IS COMPLETE.
C       IF YES, ICHECK=0; IF NO, ICHECK=1.
C       MISSING VALUES ARE CODED "-5.0" !!
C
      REAL*8 X(1)
      ICHECK=1
      DO 1 I=1,NVAR
      IF(X(I).EQ.-5.DO)GOTO2
1     CONTINUE
      ICHECK=0
2     RETURN
      END
```

```
      SUBROUTINE LOGI08(X,NVAR,LIST,WT,NOBS,TOTWT,XBAR,SSQ)
C     *****************************************************
C
C       ALGORITHM AS12 (MODIFIED) JRSS (SERIES C) 17, 1968.
C
C       INPUT TO THIS ROUTINE CONSISTS OF A SET OF VARIATE
C       VALUES X(LIST(1)),...,X(LIST(NVAR)) AND A WEIGHT WT.
C       THESE ARE USED TO UPDATE THE NUMBER OF OBSERVATIONS,
C       THE TOTAL WEIGHT,THE MEANS AND THE CORRECTED SUMS OF SQUARES.
C       IF NOBS=0 ON ENTRY,TOTWT AND SSQ ARE CLEARED.
C
      IMPLICIT REAL*8(A-H,O-Z)
      DIMENSION X(1),LIST(1),XBAR(1),SSQ(1)
      IF(NOBS.NE.0)GOTO2
      TOTWT=WT
      DO 1 I=1,NVAR
      II=LIST(I)
      SSQ(I)=0.D0
1     XBAR(I)=X(II)
      IF(WT.NE.0.D0)NOBS=1
      GOTO4
2     SW=TOTWT+WT
      IF(WT.EQ.0.D0)GOTO4
      F=WT/SW
      I=NVAR
3     II=LIST(I)
      D=(X(II)-XBAR(I))*F
      XBAR(I)=XBAR(I)+D
      SSQ(I)=SSQ(I)+D*TOTWT*D/F
      I=I-1
      IF(I.NE.0)GOTO3
      TOTWT=SW
      NOBS=NOBS+1
4     RETURN
      END


      FUNCTION DFLOAT(N)
C     ******************
C
C       TRANSFORM AN INTEGER INTO DOUBLE PRECISION REAL VARIABLE
C
      REAL*8 DFLOAT
      DFLOAT=N
      RETURN
      END

      FUNCTION INDICE (I,J)
C     *********************
C
C       DETERMINES THE INDEX (I,J) OF A SYMMETRIC MATRIX
C       HELD IN ONE-DIMENSIONAL FORM.
```

```
C
      IF(I.GE.J)GOTO1
      INDICE=I+J*(J-1)/2
      RETURN
1     INDICE=J+I*(I-1)/2
      RETURN
      END


      FUNCTION PRCHI2(X,NU,IFAULT)
C     ****************************
C
C        EVALUATES THE AREA FROM X TO PLUS INFINITY UNDER
C        A CHI-SQUARED DISTRIBUTION WITH NU DEGREES OF FREEDOM.
C
      IMPLICIT REAL*8(A-H,O-Z)
      PRCHI2=-5.DO
      IFAULT=3
      IF(X.LT.O.DO.OR.NU.LT.1)RETURN
      XX=X/2.DO
      P=DFLOAT(NU)/2.DO
      A=PRGAMA(XX,P,IFAULT)
      IF(IFAULT.GT.O)RETURN
      PRCHI2=1.DO-A
      RETURN
      END


      FUNCTION PRGAMA(X,P,IFAULT)
C     ***************************
C
C       ALGORITHM AS32 JRSS (SERIES C) 1970 VOL.19,3
C       COMPUTES INCOMPLETE GAMMA RATIO FOR POSITIVE VALUES
C       OF ARGUMENTS X AND P.
C
C       IFAULT=1,IF P.LE.0,ELSE 2,IF X.LT.0,ELSE 0
C       USES SERIES EXPANSION,IF P.GT.X OR X LE.1,
C       CONTINUED FRACTION APPROXIMATION,OTHERWISE.
C
      IMPLICIT REAL*8(A-H,O-Z)
      DIMENSION PN(6)
C
C       DEFINE ACCURACY AND INITIALIZE
C
      G=DLGAMA(P)
      ACU=1.D-8
      OFLO=1.D30
      CONST=-100.DO
      GIN=0.DO
      IFAULT=0
C
C       TEST FOR ADMISSIBILITY OF ARGUMENTS
```

```
C
      IF(P.LE.0.D0)IFAULT=1
      IF(X.LT.0.D0)IFAULT=2
      IF(IFAULT.GT.0.OR. X.EQ.0.D0)GOTO50
      EXPOS=P*DLOG(X)-X-G
      FACTOR=0.D0
      IF(EXPOS.GT.CONST)FACTOR=DEXP(EXPOS)
      IF(X.GT.1.D0.AND.X.GE.P)GOTO30
C
C       CALCULATION BY SERIES EXPANSION
C
      GIN=1.D0
      TERM=1.D0
      RN=P
20    RN=RN+1.D0
      TERM=TERM*X/RN
      GIN=GIN+TERM
      IF(TERM.GT.ACU)GOTO20
      GIN=GIN*FACTOR/P
      GOTO50
C
C       CALCULATION BY CONTINUED FRACTION
C
30    A=1.D0-P
      B=A+X+1.D0
      TERM=0.D0
      PN(1)=1.D0
      PN(2)=X
      PN(3)=X+1.D0
      PN(4)=X*B
      GIN=PN(3)/PN(4)
32    A=A+1.D0
      B=B+2.D0
      TERM=TERM+1.D0
      AN=A*TERM
      DO 33 I=1,2
33    PN(I+4)=B*PN(I+2)-AN*PN(I)
      IF(PN(6).EQ.0.D0)GOTO35
      RN=PN(5)/PN(6)
      DIF=DABS(GIN-RN)
      IF(DIF.GT.ACU)GOTO34
      IF(DIF.LE.ACU*RN)GOTO42
34    GIN=RN
35    DO 36 I=1,4
36    PN(I)=PN(I+2)
      IF(DABS(PN(5)).LT.OFLO)GOTO32
      DO 41 I=1,4
41    PN(I)=PN(I)/OFLO
      GOTO32
42    GIN=1.D0-FACTOR*GIN
C
50    PRGAMA=GIN
```

```
      RETURN
      END



      FUNCTION DLGAMA(Y)
C     ******************
C
C       THIS FUNCTION CALCULATES THE NATURAL LOGARITHM OF GAMMA(X)
C       FOR EVERY X>0 (STIRLING FORMULA).
C
C       REF: PIKE AND HILL, COMMUN. A.C.M., 9, ALGORITHM 291.
C
      IMPLICIT REAL*8(A-H,O-Z)
      X=Y
      DLGAMA=0.D0
      IF(X.EQ.1.D0.OR.X.EQ.2.D0)GOTO3
      C1=0.918938533204673
      C2=-0.000595238095238
      C3=0.000793650793651
      C4=0.002777777777778
      C5=0.083333333333333
C
      IF(X.GE.7.D0)GOTO10
      F=1.D0
      Z=X-1.D0
1     Z=Z+1.D0
      IF(Z.GE.7.D0)GOTO2
      X=Z
      F=F*Z
      GOTO1
C
2     X=X+1.0D0
      F=-DLOG(F)
      GOTO20
C
10    F=0.D0
20    Z=1.D0/X**2.D0
      DLGAMA=F+(X-0.5D0)*DLOG(X)-X+C1+
     * (((C2*Z+C3)*Z-C4)*Z+C5)/X
3     RETURN
      END
```

Output: Discriminant Analysis and Likelihood Ratio

```
MULTIPLE GROUP LOGISTIC DISCRIMINANT ANALYSIS
*********************************************

DATE ... 19-AUG-86
TIME ... 21:52:03

OUTPUT FROM MAIN PROGRAM - L O G D I S

  DISCRIMINATION BETWEEN:
  ***********************

       GROUP: 1    N= 57     PRIOR= 0.40     ACUTE VIRAL HEPATITIS
       GROUP: 2    N= 44     PRIOR= 0.31     PERSISTENT CHRONIC HEPATITIS
       GROUP: 3    N= 40     PRIOR= 0.28     AGRESSIVE CHRONIC HEPATITIS

       TOTAL NO. OF OBSERVATIONS = 141

  VARIABLES STUDIED
  *****************

       NUMBER   OVERALL MEAN    OVERALL S.D.     NAME

          1           189.08          269.251    AST
          2           340.82          359.629    ALT
          3            15.51           15.918    GLDH

  MATRIX OF MEAN VALUES
  *********************
     COLUMNS=GROUPS
     ROWS=VARIABLES

              1              2              3
  1       237.0702        59.3182       263.4250
  2       608.1754       106.5909       217.4750
  3        13.8947         7.2727        26.8750

  MATRIX OF STANDARD DEVIATIONS
  *****************************
         COLUMNS=GROUPS
         ROWS=VARIABLES

              1              2              3
  1       165.8143        73.4637       432.1824
  2       332.5551       122.6463       326.9832
  3         5.6842         3.7748        25.1918

DATABASE INFORMATION
********************

FILE NAME = HEPATIC.DAT
FORMAT USED = (A6,I4,3F10.0)
```

```
LOGISTIC DISCRIMINANT ANALYSIS
MAXIMUM LIKELIHOOD ESTIMATION
*****************************

PARAMETERS OF THE PROBLEM

NO. OF GROUPS = 3      NO. OF VARIABLES =  3     TOTAL NO. OF OBS =141
H-INV CYCLE = 1

GROUP 1      N =  57     PRIOR = 0.40
GROUP 2      N =  44     PRIOR = 0.31
GROUP 3      N =  40     PRIOR = 0.28

ITYP = 0: MIXTURE SAMPLING SCHEME
          PRIORS ARE COMPUTED FROM THE SAMPLE

ISDX = 0: ORIGINAL MATRIX OF DATA

ITERATION  0   INVERSION  0

INITIAL MATRIX OF COEFFICIENTS B

             1              2
0         0.0000         0.0000
1         0.0000         0.0000
2         0.0000         0.0000
3         0.0000         0.0000


NEWTON-RAPHSON ITERATIVE PROCEDURE


IT =  1   LOG-LIK = -154.904333
IT =  2   LOG-LIK =  -91.291108
IT =  3   LOG-LIK =  -73.606262
IT =  4   LOG-LIK =  -66.376777
IT =  5   LOG-LIK =  -64.248211
IT =  6   LOG-LIK =  -63.990772
IT =  7   LOG-LIK =  -63.984967
IT =  8   LOG-LIK =  -63.984963

MAXIMUM ATTAINED AFTER  8 ITERATIONS:  MAX LOG-LIK =  -63.984967

ITERATION  8   INVERSION  8

FINAL MATRIX OF COEFFICIENTS B

             1              2
0         0.8599         3.9321
1        -0.0232        -0.0206
2         0.0235         0.0130
3        -0.2108        -0.2981
```

MATRIX OF STD-ERRORS OF COEFFICIENTS SEB

	1	2
0	0.8574	0.7953
1	0.0071	0.0081
2	0.0056	0.0054
3	0.0742	0.0738

MATRIX OF Z-SCORES: ZB=B/SEB

	1	2
0	1.0028	4.9440
1	-3.2806	-2.5344
2	4.1660	2.3908
3	-2.8393	-4.0408

ASYMPTOTIC DISPERSION MATRIX OF COEFFICIENTS

	10	11	12	13	20
10	0.7352				
11	-0.0007	0.0000			
12	0.0005	-0.0000	0.0000		
13	-0.0443	0.0001	-0.0002	0.0055	
20	0.4289	-0.0005	0.0003	-0.0244	0.6325
21	-0.0012	0.0000	-0.0000	0.0001	-0.0016
22	0.0010	-0.0000	0.0000	-0.0002	0.0006
23	-0.0295	0.0001	-0.0001	0.0029	-0.0428

	21	22	23
21	0.0001		
22	-0.0000	0.0000	
23	-0.0000	-0.0001	0.0054

FINAL CLASSIFICATION MATRIX OF OBSERVATIONS
COLUMNS=TRUE GROUPS
ROWS=ALLOCATED GROUPS

	1	2	3
1	49	2	1
2	6	40	6
3	2	2	33
TOTAL	57	44	40

EFFECTIVENESS - CHI-SQUARE: 178.55 DF: 6 PROB: 0.0000D+00

```
MATRIX OF ALLOCATION AND PROBABILITIES
**************************************

I   NPAT       GROUP          GROUP PROB
           TRUE   ALLOC        1          2          3


 1    1      1      1        0.96       0.04       0.00
 2    2      1      1        0.63       0.18       0.19
 3    3      1      1        0.61       0.29       0.10
 4    4      1      2        0.16       0.72       0.12
 5    5      1      1        0.81       0.18       0.01
 6    6      1      1        0.79       0.21       0.00
 7    7      1      1        0.87       0.09       0.04
 8    8      1      1        0.96       0.04       0.00
 9    9      1      1        0.87       0.13       0.00
10   10      1      1        0.92       0.08       0.00
11   11      1      1        0.98       0.02       0.00
12   12      1      1        0.52       0.47       0.01
13   13      1      3        0.41       0.00       0.58
14   14      1      1        1.00       0.00       0.00
15   15      1      1        0.67       0.31       0.02
16   16      1      1        1.00       0.00       0.00
17   17      1      1        0.98       0.01       0.00
18   18      1      2        0.29       0.70       0.01
19   19      1      1        1.00       0.00       0.00
20   20      1      1        0.82       0.17       0.01
21   21      1      1        0.93       0.07       0.00
22   22      1      1        0.95       0.05       0.00
23   23      1      1        0.54       0.09       0.38
24   24      1      1        0.99       0.01       0.00
25   25      1      1        0.98       0.02       0.00
26   26      1      1        1.00       0.00       0.00
27   27      1      1        0.96       0.04       0.00
28   28      1      1        1.00       0.00       0.00
29   29      1      1        0.72       0.22       0.06
30   30      1      1        0.86       0.12       0.03
31   31      1      1        0.99       0.01       0.00
32   32      1      1        1.00       0.00       0.00
33   33      1      2        0.25       0.71       0.03
34   34      1      1        0.99       0.01       0.00
35   35      1      1        1.00       0.00       0.00
36   36      1      1        1.00       0.00       0.00
37   37      1      1        0.80       0.19       0.01
38    1      1      1        0.99       0.01       0.00
39    2      1      1        0.92       0.08       0.00
40    3      1      1        0.98       0.02       0.00
41    4      1      1        1.00       0.00       0.00
42    5      1      1        0.57       0.11       0.32
43    6      1      2        0.37       0.41       0.22
```

44	7	1	1	1.00	0.00	0.00
45	8	1	1	1.00	0.00	0.00
46	9	1	1	1.00	0.00	0.00
47	10	1	3	0.18	0.01	0.81
48	11	1	1	0.99	0.00	0.01
49	12	1	1	0.95	0.04	0.01
50	13	1	1	0.97	0.03	0.00
51	14	1	1	1.00	0.00	0.00
52	15	1	1	0.97	0.03	0.00
53	16	1	1	0.94	0.03	0.03
54	17	1	2	0.47	0.48	0.05
55	18	1	1	1.00	0.00	0.00
56	19	1	1	0.69	0.03	0.28
57	20	1	2	0.43	0.43	0.14
58	1	2	3	0.27	0.03	0.70
59	2	2	2	0.09	0.82	0.08
60	3	2	2	0.20	0.73	0.07
61	4	2	2	0.21	0.67	0.12
62	5	2	2	0.10	0.85	0.05
63	6	2	2	0.10	0.81	0.09
64	7	2	2	0.11	0.65	0.24
65	8	2	2	0.12	0.74	0.15
66	9	2	2	0.16	0.70	0.14
67	10	2	2	0.16	0.72	0.12
68	11	2	2	0.10	0.84	0.06
69	12	2	2	0.08	0.87	0.05
70	13	2	2	0.08	0.86	0.06
71	14	2	2	0.20	0.70	0.10
72	15	2	2	0.08	0.86	0.06
73	16	2	2	0.11	0.83	0.05
74	17	2	2	0.11	0.80	0.09
75	18	2	2	0.08	0.88	0.04
76	19	2	2	0.11	0.77	0.11
77	20	2	1	0.73	0.08	0.19
78	21	2	2	0.09	0.84	0.07
79	22	2	2	0.13	0.82	0.05
80	23	2	2	0.13	0.78	0.09
81	24	2	2	0.15	0.74	0.11
82	25	2	2	0.09	0.77	0.13
83	26	2	2	0.08	0.83	0.08
84	27	2	2	0.11	0.81	0.09
85	28	2	2	0.10	0.79	0.11
86	29	2	2	0.09	0.79	0.12
87	30	2	2	0.08	0.87	0.05
88	31	2	2	0.11	0.78	0.10
89	32	2	3	0.07	0.23	0.70
90	33	2	2	0.10	0.87	0.03
91	34	2	2	0.10	0.76	0.14
92	35	2	2	0.10	0.61	0.30
93	36	2	2	0.48	0.51	0.01

94	37	2	1	0.99	0.01	0.00
95	38	2	2	0.13	0.77	0.10
96	39	2	2	0.37	0.56	0.07
97	40	2	2	0.22	0.54	0.24
98	41	2	2	0.08	0.86	0.06
99	42	2	2	0.21	0.53	0.26
100	43	2	2	0.17	0.58	0.26
101	44	2	2	0.12	0.79	0.09
102	1	3	3	0.00	0.00	1.00
103	2	3	3	0.11	0.14	0.75
104	3	3	3	0.15	0.20	0.65
105	4	3	3	0.31	0.13	0.56
106	5	3	3	0.00	0.00	1.00
107	6	3	2	0.09	0.74	0.17
108	7	3	3	0.03	0.42	0.55
109	8	3	3	0.08	0.14	0.78
110	9	3	2	0.09	0.63	0.28
111	10	3	3	0.08	0.39	0.52
112	11	3	3	0.06	0.01	0.93
113	12	3	3	0.02	0.08	0.90
114	13	3	3	0.00	0.00	1.00
115	14	3	3	0.13	0.34	0.52
116	15	3	2	0.07	0.83	0.11
117	16	3	3	0.00	0.00	0.99
118	17	3	3	0.00	0.00	1.00
119	18	3	3	0.04	0.04	0.93
120	19	3	3	0.02	0.04	0.94
121	20	3	2	0.09	0.63	0.28
122	21	3	2	0.08	0.60	0.32
123	22	3	3	0.03	0.17	0.80
124	23	3	2	0.16	0.53	0.32
125	24	3	3	0.06	0.07	0.87
126	25	3	3	0.00	0.00	1.00
127	26	3	3	0.04	0.02	0.93
128	27	3	3	0.02	0.07	0.91
129	28	3	3	0.08	0.14	0.78
130	29	3	3	0.00	0.00	0.99
131	30	3	3	0.01	0.04	0.96
132	31	3	3	0.05	0.01	0.93
133	32	3	3	0.00	0.00	1.00
134	33	3	3	0.00	0.00	1.00
135	34	3	3	0.00	0.00	1.00
136	35	3	1	1.00	0.00	0.00
137	36	3	3	0.01	0.00	0.99
138	37	3	3	0.00	0.00	1.00
139	38	3	3	0.00	0.00	1.00
140	39	3	3	0.00	0.00	1.00
141	40	3	3	0.00	0.00	1.00

MATRIX OF OBSERVATIONS
****

I	NPAT	GROUP	VAR 1	2	3
1	1	1	236.00	582.00	10.00
2	2	1	65.00	258.00	20.00
3	3	1	59.00	244.00	16.00
4	4	1	92.00	120.00	6.00
5	5	1	99.00	352.00	13.00
6	6	1	87.00	380.00	7.00
7	7	1	202.00	429.00	15.00
8	8	1	208.00	539.00	14.00
9	9	1	105.00	465.00	4.00
10	10	1	95.00	442.00	13.00
11	11	1	215.00	570.00	17.00
12	12	1	101.00	277.00	6.00
13	13	1	454.00	639.00	27.00
14	14	1	308.00	1243.00	9.00
15	15	1	82.00	294.00	11.00
16	16	1	196.00	760.00	18.00
17	17	1	141.00	550.00	24.00
18	18	1	73.00	201.00	3.00
19	19	1	569.00	1354.00	24.00
20	20	1	125.00	390.00	10.00
21	21	1	77.00	480.00	9.00
22	22	1	78.00	495.00	12.00
23	23	1	165.00	330.00	21.00
24	24	1	214.00	680.00	10.00
25	25	1	141.00	539.00	21.00
26	26	1	220.00	990.00	18.00
27	27	1	127.00	480.00	18.00
28	28	1	324.00	936.00	2.00
29	29	1	149.00	334.00	13.00
30	30	1	270.00	465.00	10.00
31	31	1	178.00	660.00	12.00
32	32	1	202.00	693.00	19.00
33	33	1	56.00	158.00	6.00
34	34	1	129.00	704.00	14.00
35	35	1	682.00	1595.00	20.00
36	36	1	290.00	987.00	20.00
37	37	1	61.00	327.00	14.00
38	1	1	289.00	693.00	9.00
39	2	1	133.00	470.00	11.00
40	3	1	170.00	620.00	13.00
41	4	1	550.00	1034.00	18.00
42	5	1	313.00	414.00	13.00
43	6	1	166.00	239.00	10.00
44	7	1	340.00	840.00	12.00
45	8	1	660.00	1287.00	21.00
46	9	1	321.00	1254.00	18.00

47	10	1	401.00	492.00	22.00
48	11	1	665.00	970.00	14.00
49	12	1	242.00	528.00	16.00
50	13	1	339.00	627.00	11.00
51	14	1	372.00	910.00	19.00
52	15	1	165.00	584.00	9.00
53	16	1	385.00	610.00	13.00
54	17	1	152.00	270.00	7.00
55	18	1	605.00	1199.00	16.00
56	19	1	247.00	452.00	23.00
57	20	1	123.00	231.00	11.00
58	1	2	473.00	506.00	13.00
59	2	2	40.00	52.00	5.00
60	3	2	53.00	123.00	7.00
61	4	2	76.00	133.00	8.00
62	5	2	31.00	63.00	4.00
63	6	2	32.00	56.00	6.00
64	7	2	50.00	59.00	9.00
65	8	2	56.00	72.00	7.00
66	9	2	39.00	87.00	9.00
67	10	2	46.00	95.00	8.00
68	11	2	29.00	57.00	5.00
69	12	2	40.00	50.00	3.00
70	13	2	29.00	44.00	4.00
71	14	2	77.00	132.00	7.00
72	15	2	28.00	44.00	4.00
73	16	2	28.00	68.00	5.00
74	17	2	34.00	58.00	6.00
75	18	2	24.00	42.00	3.00
76	19	2	34.00	61.00	7.00
77	20	2	119.00	345.00	23.00
78	21	2	26.00	41.00	5.00
79	22	2	39.00	84.00	5.00
80	23	2	30.00	70.00	7.00
81	24	2	35.00	81.00	8.00
82	25	2	29.00	41.00	7.00
83	26	2	31.00	38.00	5.00
84	27	2	31.00	56.00	6.00
85	28	2	23.00	43.00	7.00
86	29	2	38.00	40.00	6.00
87	30	2	22.00	42.00	4.00
88	31	2	26.00	57.00	7.00
89	32	2	26.00	42.00	17.00
90	33	2	35.00	72.00	3.00
91	34	2	42.00	53.00	7.00
92	35	2	41.00	47.00	10.00
93	36	2	64.00	260.00	5.00
94	37	2	212.00	660.00	14.00
95	38	2	83.00	101.00	5.00
96	39	2	64.00	185.00	10.00

97	40	2	121.00	159.00	9.00
98	41	2	29.00	42.00	4.00
99	42	2	129.00	163.00	9.00
100	43	2	76.00	109.00	10.00
101	44	2	20.00	57.00	7.00
102	1	3	135.00	118.00	50.00
103	2	3	75.00	125.00	19.00
104	3	3	120.00	163.00	16.00
105	4	3	99.00	224.00	21.00
106	5	3	112.00	93.00	52.00
107	6	3	71.00	61.00	6.00
108	7	3	144.00	42.00	6.00
109	8	3	52.00	86.00	19.00
110	9	3	46.00	40.00	9.00
111	10	3	49.00	51.00	13.00
112	11	3	266.00	316.00	23.00
113	12	3	52.00	30.00	19.00
114	13	3	139.00	132.00	47.00
115	14	3	50.00	89.00	15.00
116	15	3	53.00	31.00	4.00
117	16	3	216.00	146.00	24.00
118	17	3	246.00	114.00	24.00
119	18	3	74.00	115.00	24.00
120	19	3	137.00	94.00	18.00
121	20	3	70.00	53.00	8.00
122	21	3	80.00	55.00	8.00
123	22	3	115.00	58.00	13.00
124	23	3	119.00	132.00	9.00
125	24	3	222.00	204.00	15.00
126	25	3	660.00	418.00	28.00
127	26	3	159.00	197.00	23.00
128	27	3	86.00	52.00	18.00
129	28	3	103.00	118.00	17.00
130	29	3	91.00	52.00	27.00
131	30	3	110.00	32.00	18.00
132	31	3	192.00	255.00	25.00
133	32	3	540.00	184.00	160.00
134	33	3	490.00	425.00	41.00
135	34	3	2298.00	1310.00	43.00
136	35	3	858.00	1551.00	29.00
137	36	3	87.00	139.00	34.00
138	37	3	184.00	112.00	28.00
139	38	3	100.00	94.00	52.00
140	39	3	1561.00	979.00	31.00
141	40	3	276.00	209.00	39.00

```
MATRIX OF SCORES
****************
```

I	NPAT	GROUP	SCORES 1	2
1	1	1	6.94	3.64
2	2	1	1.19	-0.02
3	3	1	1.85	1.11
4	4	1	0.28	1.81
5	5	1	4.09	2.58
6	6	1	6.29	4.98
7	7	1	3.09	0.86
8	8	1	5.74	2.46
9	9	1	8.50	6.60
10	10	1	6.29	3.83
11	11	1	5.67	1.83
12	12	1	3.76	3.65
13	13	1	-0.35	-5.18
14	14	1	21.00	11.02
15	15	1	3.54	2.78
16	16	1	10.36	4.38
17	17	1	5.44	1.00
18	18	1	3.25	4.14
19	19	1	14.40	2.61
20	20	1	5.01	3.43
21	21	1	8.45	5.89
22	22	1	8.14	5.16
23	23	1	0.36	-1.45
24	24	1	9.75	5.36
25	25	1	5.82	1.76
26	26	1	15.21	6.87
27	27	1	5.39	2.17
28	28	1	14.90	8.80
29	29	1	2.51	1.32
30	30	1	3.41	1.42
31	31	1	9.70	5.24
32	32	1	8.44	3.09
33	33	1	2.01	3.04
34	34	1	11.44	6.23
35	35	1	18.28	4.60
36	36	1	13.09	4.79
37	37	1	4.17	2.74
38	1	1	8.53	4.28
39	2	1	6.49	4.01
40	3	1	8.73	4.59
41	4	1	8.59	0.65
42	5	1	0.59	-1.02
43	6	1	0.52	0.63
44	7	1	10.17	4.24
45	8	1	11.35	0.77
46	9	1	19.06	8.21

47	10	1	-1.52	-4.50
48	11	1	5.27	-1.36
49	12	1	4.27	1.02
50	13	1	5.40	1.80
51	14	1	9.60	2.40
52	15	1	8.85	5.42
53	16	1	3.52	0.04
54	17	1	2.20	2.22
55	18	1	11.61	2.25
56	19	1	0.90	-2.15
57	20	1	1.11	1.11
58	1	2	-0.96	-3.12
59	2	2	0.10	2.29
60	3	2	1.04	2.35
61	4	2	0.53	1.71
62	5	2	0.78	2.92
63	6	2	0.17	2.21
64	7	2	-0.81	0.98
65	8	2	-0.22	1.63
66	9	2	0.10	1.57
67	10	2	0.34	1.83
68	11	2	0.47	2.58
69	12	2	0.47	2.86
70	13	2	0.38	2.71
71	14	2	0.70	1.97
72	15	2	0.40	2.73
73	16	2	0.75	2.75
74	17	2	0.17	2.20
75	18	2	0.66	3.09
76	19	2	0.03	1.94
77	20	2	1.35	-0.90
78	21	2	0.17	2.44
79	22	2	0.87	2.73
80	23	2	0.33	2.14
81	24	2	0.26	1.88
82	25	2	-0.32	1.78
83	26	2	-0.02	2.30
84	27	2	0.19	2.23
85	28	2	-0.14	1.93
86	29	2	-0.35	1.88
87	30	2	0.49	2.83
88	31	2	0.12	2.05
89	32	2	-2.34	-1.13
90	33	2	1.11	3.25
91	34	2	-0.34	1.67
92	35	2	-1.09	0.72
93	36	2	4.43	4.49
94	37	2	8.49	3.95
95	38	2	0.25	2.04
96	39	2	1.61	2.03

97	40	2	-0.11	0.82
98	41	2	0.33	2.69
99	42	2	-0.20	0.71
100	43	2	-0.45	0.80
101	44	2	0.26	2.17
102	1	3	-10.04	-12.22
103	2	3	-1.95	-1.66
104	3	3	-1.47	-1.20
105	4	3	-0.60	-1.46
106	5	3	-10.51	-12.67
107	6	3	-0.62	1.47
108	7	3	-2.75	-0.28
109	8	3	-2.33	-1.69
110	9	3	-1.16	0.82
111	10	3	-1.82	-0.29
112	11	3	-2.73	-4.30
113	12	3	-3.65	-2.41
114	13	3	-9.17	-11.23
115	14	3	-1.37	-0.42
116	15	3	-0.48	2.05
117	16	3	-5.78	-5.78
118	17	3	-7.22	-6.81
119	18	3	-3.21	-3.26
120	19	3	-3.90	-3.04
121	20	3	-1.20	0.79
122	21	3	-1.39	0.61
123	22	3	-3.18	-1.56
124	23	3	-0.70	0.51
125	24	3	-2.66	-2.47
126	25	3	-10.52	-12.58
127	26	3	-3.05	-3.64
128	27	3	-3.71	-2.53
129	28	3	-2.34	-1.73
130	29	3	-5.72	-5.32
131	30	3	-4.73	-3.28
132	31	3	-2.87	-4.17
133	32	3	-41.05	-52.49
134	33	3	-9.16	-12.87
135	34	3	-30.69	-39.21
136	35	3	11.27	-2.27
137	36	3	-5.06	-6.19
138	37	3	-6.68	-6.75
139	38	3	-10.21	-12.41
140	39	3	-18.86	-24.75
141	40	3	-8.85	-10.67

```
MULTIPLE GROUP LOGISTIC DISCRIMINANT ANALYSIS
*********************************************

DATE ... 19-AUG-86
TIME ... 21:38:12

OUTPUT FROM MAIN PROGRAM - L O G D I S

  DISCRIMINATION BETWEEN:
  ***********************

       GROUP: 1  N= 57    PRIOR= 1.00   ACUTE VIRAL HEPATITIS (GROUP D)
       GROUP: 2  N= 84    PRIOR= 1.00   CHRONIC HEPATITIS (GROUP DBAR)

       TOTAL NO. OF OBSERVATIONS = 141


  VARIABLES STUDIED
  *****************

       NUMBER   OVERALL MEAN    OVERALL S.D.     NAME

          2            340.82         359.629    ALT


  MATRIX OF MEAN VALUES
  *********************
     COLUMNS=GROUPS
     ROWS=VARIABLES

             1             2
  2      608.1754      159.3929


  MATRIX OF STANDARD DEVIATIONS
  *****************************
         COLUMNS=GROUPS
         ROWS=VARIABLES

             1             2
  2      332.5551      247.2555



DATABASE INFORMATION
********************

FILE NAME = HEPATIC.DAT
FORMAT USED = (A6,I4,3F10.0)
```

```
LOGISTIC DISCRIMINANT ANALYSIS
MAXIMUM LIKELIHOOD ESTIMATION
*****************************

PARAMETERS OF THE PROBLEM

NO. OF GROUPS = 2      NO. OF VARIABLES =  1     TOTAL NO. OF OBS =141
H-INV CYCLE = 1


GROUP 1      N =  57      PRIOR = 1.00
GROUP 2      N =  84      PRIOR = 1.00


ITYP = 1: SEPARATE SAMPLING SCHEME
          PRIORS ARE GIVEN BY USER
          ADJUSTMENT OF MLE REQUIRED FOR INDEPENDENT TERMS


ATTENTION: BOTH PRIORS ARE EQUAL TO ONE
*********

     - PROGRAM "LOGISD" IS USED FOR COMPUTING
       THE LIKELIHOOD RATIO FUNCTION BETWEEN
       GROUP1 (D) AND GROUP2 (DBAR):

               L(X) = EXP(BO + B.X)

       WHERE BO AND B ARE GIVEN IN FINAL MATRIX
       OF COEFFICIENTS B BELOW

     - IN THE CLASSIFICATION MATRIX BELOW,
       COLUMNS ARE GROUPS D AND DBAR, WHILE
       ROWS ARE L>1 AND L<1, RESPECTIVELY

  ISDX = 0: ORIGINAL MATRIX OF DATA

ITERATION  0   INVERSION  0

INITIAL MATRIX OF COEFFICIENTS B

           1
0        0.0000
1        0.0000


NEWTON-RAPHSON ITERATIVE PROCEDURE

IT =  1   LOG-LIK =  -97.733752
IT =  2   LOG-LIK =  -65.911162
IT =  3   LOG-LIK =  -61.783395
```

```
IT =  4   LOG-LIK =  -61.350458
IT =  5   LOG-LIK =  -61.344601
IT =  6   LOG-LIK =  -61.344600

MAXIMUM ATTAINED AFTER  6 ITERATIONS:  MAX LOG-LIK =  -61.344601


ITERATION  6   INVERSION  6

FINAL MATRIX OF COEFFICIENTS B

            1
0        -1.9533
1         0.0062


MATRIX OF STD-ERRORS OF COEFFICIENTS SEB

            1
0         0.3364
1         0.0011


MATRIX OF Z-SCORES: ZB=B/SEB

            1
0        -5.8065
1         5.7700


ASYMPTOTIC DISPERSION MATRIX OF COEFFICIENTS

           10             11
10        0.1132
11       -0.0003         0.0000


FINAL CLASSIFICATION MATRIX OF OBSERVATIONS
            COLUMNS=TRUE GROUPS
            ROWS=ALLOCATED GROUPS

            1        2

    1      47        9
    2      10       75

  TOTAL    57       84

EFFECTIVENESS - CHI-SQUARE:   67.58   DF:  1   PROB:  0.2082D-15

DATE ... 19-AUG-86
TIME ... 21:38:12
```

```
MULTIPLE GROUP LOGISTIC DISCRIMINANT ANALYSIS
*********************************************

DATE ... 19-AUG-86
TIME ... 21:38:12

OUTPUT FROM MAIN PROGRAM - L O G D I S

  DISCRIMINATION BETWEEN:
  ***********************

      GROUP: 1   N= 57   PRIOR= 1.00   ACUTE VIRAL HEPATITIS (GROUP D)
      GROUP: 2   N= 84   PRIOR= 1.00   CHRONIC HEPATITIS (GROUP DBAR)

      TOTAL NO. OF OBSERVATIONS = 141


  VARIABLES STUDIED
  *****************

      NUMBER   OVERALL MEAN   OVERALL S.D.    NAME

         1           189.08        269.251    AST
         2           340.82        359.629    ALT


  MATRIX OF MEAN VALUES
  *********************
     COLUMNS=GROUPS
     ROWS=VARIABLES

              1              2
  1      237.0702       156.5119
  2      608.1754       159.3929


  MATRIX OF STANDARD DEVIATIONS
  *****************************
         COLUMNS=GROUPS
         ROWS=VARIABLES

              1              2
  1      165.8143       317.9266
  2      332.5551       247.2555


DATABASE INFORMATION
********************

FILE NAME = HEPATIC.DAT
FORMAT USED = (A6,I4,3F10.0)
```

```
LOGISTIC DISCRIMINANT ANALYSIS
MAXIMUM LIKELIHOOD ESTIMATION
*****************************

PARAMETERS OF THE PROBLEM

NO. OF GROUPS = 2      NO. OF VARIABLES =  2     TOTAL NO. OF OBS =141
H-INV CYCLE = 1


GROUP 1      N =  57      PRIOR = 1.00
GROUP 2      N =  84      PRIOR = 1.00


ITYP = 1: SEPARATE SAMPLING SCHEME
          PRIORS ARE GIVEN BY USER
          ADJUSTMENT OF MLE REQUIRED FOR INDEPENDENT TERMS


ATTENTION: BOTH PRIORS ARE EQUAL TO ONE
*********

    - PROGRAM "LOGISD" IS USED FOR COMPUTING
      THE LIKELIHOOD RATIO FUNCTION BETWEEN
      GROUP1 (D) AND GROUP2 (DBAR):

              L(X) = EXP(BO + B.X)

      WHERE BO AND B ARE GIVEN IN FINAL MATRIX
      OF COEFFICIENTS B BELOW

    - IN THE CLASSIFICATION MATRIX BELOW,
      COLUMNS ARE GROUPS D AND DBAR, WHILE
      ROWS ARE L>1 AND L<1, RESPECTIVELY

ISDX = 0: ORIGINAL MATRIX OF DATA

ITERATION  0   INVERSION  0

INITIAL MATRIX OF COEFFICIENTS B

           1
0        0.0000
1        0.0000
2        0.0000

NEWTON-RAPHSON ITERATIVE PROCEDURE

IT =  1   LOG-LIK =  -97.733752
IT =  2   LOG-LIK =  -54.165646
IT =  3   LOG-LIK =  -44.329178
IT =  4   LOG-LIK =  -41.457422
```

```
IT =  5   LOG-LIK =  -41.030924
IT =  6   LOG-LIK =  -41.018446
IT =  7   LOG-LIK =  -41.018433

MAXIMUM ATTAINED AFTER  7 ITERATIONS:  MAX LOG-LIK =  -41.018446

ITERATION  7   INVERSION  7

FINAL MATRIX OF COEFFICIENTS B

            1
0       -2.2722
1       -0.0142
2        0.0156


MATRIX OF STD-ERRORS OF COEFFICIENTS SEB

            1
0        0.4485
1        0.0044
2        0.0029


MATRIX OF Z-SCORES: ZB=B/SEB

            1
0       -5.0667
1       -3.2242
2        5.4331


ASYMPTOTIC DISPERSION MATRIX OF COEFFICIENTS

            10           11           12
10        0.2011
11       -0.0000       0.0000
12       -0.0006      -0.0000       0.0000


FINAL CLASSIFICATION MATRIX OF OBSERVATIONS
            COLUMNS=TRUE GROUPS
            ROWS=ALLOCATED GROUPS

            1       2

    1      49       4
    2       8      80

  TOTAL    57      84

EFFECTIVENESS - CHI-SQUARE:  108.23   DF:  2   PROB:  0.0000D+00
```

C. TIMSER: A PROGRAM FOR SERIAL OBSERVATIONS

Description of Program

This program for applying the homeostatic (white noise) and random walk time series models discussed in Chapter 8 is intended for equispaced data series with no missing observations. It is written in BASIC for an IBM Personal Computer with on-line printer. Input/Output statements such as Numbers 30 and 235, and later PRINT #1 statements may have to be modified for other systems. The application given here refers to the cholesterol data in Table 8.1 (Series A). Therefore, the length of series N in Statement 50 was set equal to 5, the analytical standard deviation A in Statement 135 was set to 4 (mg/100 ml), and the data themselves listed in Statement 355. Of course, these numbers would be different in another application. Student's t-values are listed for degrees of freedom 2 to 18 in Statements 345 and 350, and α (probability of error of the first kind) was set to 0.1. The output of this application is given in Table 8.1 (Series A).

Although the program appears to be retrospective following the input of N observations, it is in fact sequential and may be rerun after each new observation simply by updating the value of N and adding the new observation to the list of data. However, at least three observations are necessary to initiate the calculations.

Listing of Program (BASIC)

```
5 REM TIMSER
10 REM prog. for homeostatic and random walk models
15 DIM Z(20),X(50),M(50),S(50),S1(50),D(50),T(50)
20 DIM V(50),C(50),W(50),Y(50),H1(50),H2(50),R1(50),R2(50),E(50)
25 REM Z(I) = Student's "t" with I d.f. and prob.=.10
30 OPEN "lpt1:" FOR OUTPUT AS #1
35 FOR I=2 TO 18
```

```
40 READ Z(I)
45 NEXT I
50 N=5
55 FOR I=1 TO N
60 READ X(I)
65 NEXT I
70 M(1)=X(1)
75 Y(1)=X(1)
80 W(1)=1
85 S(1)=0
90 FOR I=2 TO N
95 M(I)=((I-1)*M(I-1)+X(I))/I
100 S(I)=((I-2)/(I-1))*S(I-1)+((M(I-1)-X(I))^2)/I
105 S1(I)=SQR(S(I))
110 D(I)=X(I)-X(I-1)
115 NEXT I
120 REM mean(t) and variance (v) of diff's.
125 T(2)=D(2)
130 V(2)=0
135 A=4
140 FOR I=3 TO N
145 T(I)=((I-2)*T(I-1)+D(I))/(I-1)
150 V(I)=((I-3)/(I-2))*V(I-1)+((T(I-1)-D(I))^2)/(I-1)
155 C(I)=(V(I)/(A^2))-2
160 IF C(I)<0,THEN 170
165 GOTO 175
170 C(I)=0
175 W(2)=(1+C(3))/(2+C(3))
180 W(I)=(W(I-1)+C(I))/(W(I-1)+C(I)+1)
185 Y(2)=W(2)*X(2)+(1-W(2))*X(1)
190 Y(I)=W(I)*X(I)+(1-W(I))*Y(I-1)
195 NEXT I
200 FOR I=4 TO N+1
205 H1(I)=M(I-1)-Z(I-2)*S1(I-1)*SQR(I/(I-1))
210 H2(I)=M(I-1)+Z(I-2)*S1(I-1)*SQR(I/(I-1))
215 R1(I)=Y(I-1)-Z(I-2)*A*SQR(W(I-1)+C(I-1)+1)
220 R2(I)=Y(I-1)+Z(I-2)*A*SQR(W(I-1)+C(I-1)+1)
225 E(I)=A*SQR(W(I-1)+C(I-1)+1)
230 NEXT I
235 PRINT #1,"i","x","mean(x)","std(x)","weight(w)"
240 PRINT #1,
245 FOR I=1 TO N
250 PRINT #1,I,X(I),M(I),S1(I),W(I)
255 NEXT I
260 PRINT #1,
265 PRINT #1,"i","pred. value","s.e. of pred. value"
270 PRINT #1,
275 FOR I=4 TO N+1
280 PRINT #1,I,Y(I-1),E(I)
285 NEXT I
```

```
290 PRINT #1,
295 PRINT #1,"i","var.diff.","c"
300 FOR I=3 TO N
305 PRINT #1,
310 PRINT #1,I,V(I),C(I)
315 NEXT I
320 PRINT #1,
325 PRINT #1,"i","h-model lowerlim","h-model upperlim",
"r-model lowerlim","r-model upperlim"
330 FOR I=4 TO N+1
335 PRINT #1,I,H1(I),H2(I),R1(I),R2(I)
340 NEXT I
345 DATA 2.92,2.35,2.13,2.02,1.94,1.90,1.86,1.83,1.81
350 DATA 1.80,1.78,1.77,1.76,1.75,1.75,1.74,1.73
355 DATA 193,195,189,204,200
360 END
```

Index

B

C

D

E

F

G

H

I

J

K

L

M